DELIBERATE PRACTICE IN
RATIONAL EMOTIVE
BEHAVIOR THERAPY

Essentials of Deliberate Practice Series
Tony Rousmaniere and Alexandre Vaz, Series Editors

Deliberate Practice in Child and Adolescent Psychotherapy
Jordan Bate, Tracy A. Prout, Tony Rousmaniere, and
Alexandre Vaz

Deliberate Practice in Cognitive Behavioral Therapy
James F. Boswell and Michael J. Constantino

Deliberate Practice in Dialectical Behavior Therapy
Tali Boritz, Shelley McMain, Alexandre Vaz, and
Tony Rousmaniere

Deliberate Practice in Emotion-Focused Therapy
Rhonda N. Goldman, Alexandre Vaz, and Tony Rousmaniere

Deliberate Practice in Motivational Interviewing
Jennifer K. Manuel, Denise Ernst, Alexandre Vaz, and
Tony Rousmaniere

Deliberate Practice in Rational Emotive Behavior Therapy
Mark D. Terjesen, Kristene A. Doyle, Raymond A. DiGiuseppe,
Alexandre Vaz, and Tony Rousmaniere

Deliberate Practice in Schema Therapy
Wendy T. Behary, Joan M. Farrell, Alexandre Vaz, and
Tony Rousmaniere

Deliberate Practice in Systemic Family Therapy
Adrian J. Blow, Ryan B. Seedall, Debra L. Miller,
Tony Rousmaniere, and Alexandre Vaz

ESSENTIALS OF DELIBERATE PRACTICE SERIES

TONY ROUSMANIERE AND ALEXANDRE VAZ, SERIES EDITORS

DELIBERATE PRACTICE IN
RATIONAL EMOTIVE BEHAVIOR THERAPY

MARK D. TERJESEN

KRISTENE A. DOYLE

RAYMOND A. DiGIUSEPPE

ALEXANDRE VAZ

TONY ROUSMANIERE

AMERICAN PSYCHOLOGICAL ASSOCIATION

Published by
American Psychological Association
750 First Street, NE
Washington, DC 20002
https://www.apa.org

Order Department
https://www.apa.org/pubs/books
order@apa.org

In the U.K., Europe, Africa, and the Middle East, copies may be ordered from Eurospan
https://www.eurospanbookstore.com/apa
info@eurospangroup.com

Typeset in Cera Pro by Circle Graphics, Inc., Reisterstown, MD

Printer: Gasch Printing, Odenton, MD
Cover Designer: Mark Karis

Library of Congress Cataloging-in-Publication Data

Names: Terjesen, Mark D. (Mark David), author. | Doyle, Kristene A., author. | DiGiuseppe, Raymond, author. | Vaz, Alexandre, author. | Rousmaniere, Tony, author.
Title: Deliberate practice in rational emotive behavior therapy / by Mark D. Terjesen, Kristene A. Doyle, Raymond A. DiGiuseppe, Alexandre Vaz, and Tony Rousmaniere.
Description: Washington, DC : American Psychological Association, [2023] | Series: Essentials of deliberate practice | Includes bibliographical references and index.
Identifiers: LCCN 2022043378 (print) | LCCN 2022043379 (ebook) | ISBN 9781433838354 (paperback) | ISBN 9781433838361 (ebook)
Subjects: LCSH: Rational emotive behavior therapy--Problems, exercises, etc. | BISAC: PSYCHOLOGY / Education & Training | PSYCHOLOGY / Psychotherapy / Counseling
Classification: LCC RC489.R3 T447 2023 (print) | LCC RC489.R3 (ebook) | DDC 616.89/14--dc23/eng/20221018
LC record available at https://lccn.loc.gov/2022043378
LC ebook record available at https://lccn.loc.gov/2022043379

https://doi.org/10.1037/0000334-000

Printed in the United States of America

10 9 8 7 6 5 4 3 2 1

We dedicate this book to our mentor, Albert Ellis, the founder of rational emotive behavior therapy (REBT) and grandfather of cognitive behavioral therapy. Al trained and taught each of us to push the science and clinical applications of REBT and always valued the importance of practice in skill development. We like to think that this book on deliberate practice and REBT is an extension of his beliefs in how to develop skills in REBT to best assist our clients.

—Mark D. Terjesen, Kristene A. Doyle, and Raymond A. DiGiuseppe

Contents

Part III   Strategies for Enhancing the Deliberate Practice Exercises   195

Series Preface

Tony Rousmaniere and Alexandre Vaz

We are pleased to introduce the Essentials of Deliberate Practice series of training books. We are developing this book series to address a specific need that we see in many psychology training programs. The issue can be illustrated by the training experiences of Mary, a hypothetical second-year graduate school trainee. Mary has learned a lot about mental health theory, research, and psychotherapy techniques. Mary is a dedicated student; she has read dozens of textbooks, written excellent papers about psychotherapy, and receives near-perfect scores on her course exams. However, when Mary sits with her clients at her practicum site, she often has trouble performing the therapy skills that she can write and talk about so clearly. Furthermore, Mary has noticed herself getting anxious when her clients express strong reactions, such as getting very emotional, hopeless, or skeptical about therapy. Sometimes this anxiety is strong enough to make Mary freeze at key moments, limiting her ability to help those clients.

During her weekly individual and group supervision, Mary's supervisor gives her advice informed by empirically supported therapies and common factor methods. The supervisor often supplements that advice by leading Mary through role-plays, recommending additional reading, or providing examples from her own work with clients. Mary, a dedicated supervisee who shares tapes of her sessions with her supervisor, is open about her challenges, carefully writes down her supervisor's advice, and reads the suggested readings. However, when Mary sits back down with her clients, she often finds that her new knowledge seems to have flown out of her head, and she is unable to enact her supervisor's advice. Mary finds this problem to be particularly acute with the clients who are emotionally evocative.

Mary's supervisor, who has received formal training in supervision, uses supervisory best practices, including the use of video to review supervisees' work. She would rate Mary's overall competence level as consistent with expectations for a trainee at Mary's developmental level. But even though Mary's overall progress is positive, she experiences some recurring problems in her work. This is true even though the supervisor is confident that she and Mary have identified the changes that Mary should make in her work.

The problem with which Mary and her supervisor are wrestling—the disconnect between her knowledge about psychotherapy and her ability to reliably perform psychotherapy—is the focus of this book series. We started this series because most therapists experience this disconnect, to one degree or another, whether they are beginning trainees or highly experienced clinicians. In truth, we are all Mary.

To address this problem, we are focusing this series on the use of deliberate practice, a method of training specifically designed for improving reliable performance of complex skills in challenging work environments (Rousmaniere, 2016, 2019; Rousmaniere et al., 2017). Deliberate practice entails experiential, repeated training with a particular skill until it becomes automatic. In the context of psychotherapy, this involves two trainees role-playing as a client and a therapist, switching roles every so often, under the guidance of a supervisor. The trainee playing the therapist reacts to client statements, ranging in difficulty from beginner to intermediate to advanced, with improvised responses that reflect fundamental therapeutic skills.

To create these books, we approached leading trainers and researchers of major therapy models with these simple instructions: Identify 10 to 12 essential skills for your therapy model where trainees often experience a disconnect between cognitive knowledge and performance ability—in other words, skills that trainees could write a good paper about but often have challenges performing, especially with challenging clients. We then collaborated with the authors to create deliberate practice exercises specifically designed to improve reliable performance of these skills and overall responsive treatment (Hatcher, 2015; Stiles et al., 1998; Stiles & Horvath, 2017). Finally, we rigorously tested these exercises with trainees and trainers at multiple sites around the world and refined them based on extensive feedback.

Each book in this series focuses on a specific therapy model, but readers will notice that most exercises in these books touch on common factor variables and facilitative interpersonal skills that researchers have identified as having the most impact on client outcome, such as empathy, verbal fluency, emotional expression, persuasiveness, and problem focus (e.g., Anderson et al., 2009; Norcross et al., 2019). Thus, the exercises in every book should help with a broad range of clients. Despite the specific theoretical model(s) from which therapists work, most therapists place a strong emphasis on pantheoretical elements of the therapeutic relationship, many of which have robust empirical support as correlates or mechanisms of client improvement (e.g., Norcross et al., 2019). We also recognize that therapy models have already-established training programs with rich histories, so we present deliberate practice not as a replacement but as an adaptable, transtheoretical training method that can be integrated into these existing programs to improve skill retention and help ensure basic competency.

About This Book

This book in the series is on rational emotive behavior therapy (REBT). REBT was developed by Albert Ellis in 1955 and is considered the pioneering and original form of cognitive behavioral therapy. The theory, and, as a result, the clinical approach, is based on the premise that negative emotional and behavioral responses are a result of unhealthy, illogical irrational beliefs held by clients (DiGiuseppe et al., 2014). Irrational beliefs are considered to be rigid and extreme in nature and inconsistent with reality (Turner, 2016), and they may reflect an overall view or philosophical belief system about oneself, others, and the world or life conditions. That is, while an individual may communicate that they believe "My partner should respect me," they may also have an underlying belief system of "Those who are important people in my life should respect me." Rational beliefs, on the other hand, are consistent with reality and are both flexible and logical in process. Clinicians help clients to understand that those irrational beliefs are not helpful in goal attainment and are inconsistent with what is true and result in emotional and/or behavioral distress. This process is accomplished through challenging or disputing those irrational beliefs. Finally, clinical work focuses on developing more functional or adaptive beliefs to replace the irrational ones to enable clients to experience healthier reactions to adverse events (D. David et al., 2018).

Training in REBT typically involves learning the theories that underlie the REBT model, observing expert practice, experiential exercises (e.g., role-playing), and supervised clinical work. The formal training offered at the Albert Ellis Institute has for more than 50 years involved direct practice and demonstration of REBT skills under the supervision of an expert REBT clinician. We see deliberate practice as an additional component designed to enhance REBT training. Deliberate practice is not intended to be the only delivery format through which REBT skills are acquired, nor is this book by itself sufficient for obtaining full competence in REBT. However, the practice of the skills set forth in this book provides trainees with the opportunity to translate their didactic learning of REBT to a simulated environment that mimics the clinical interaction, which can later be applied with actual clients. This book provides opportunities for trainees to experiment with using REBT skills with a range of client presentations and clinical scenarios and to practice what they would say and how they would say it. Our goal in writing this book is to encourage interest and engagement in REBT and support your ongoing development as REBT therapists in training.

Acknowledgments

We would like to acknowledge Rodney Goodyear for his significant contribution to starting and organizing this book series. We are grateful to Susan Reynolds, David Becker, Joe Albrecht, Elizabeth Budd, and Emily Ekle at American Psychological Association (APA) Books for providing expert guidance and insightful editing that has significantly improved the quality and accessibility of this book. We would also like to acknowledge the International Deliberate Practice Society and its members for their many contributions and support for our work. Finally, we are grateful for the invaluable support, editorial notes, and feedback from Inês Amaro.

The first three authors of this book would like to acknowledge Alex Vaz and Tony Rousmaniere, who provided guidance, support, and expert knowledge to us throughout the project, and for that we are very appreciative. We thank Brooke Catanzaro, Michelle S. Sensra, and Jessica Weiss for their valuable editorial feedback and for providing initial piloting of the exercises.

The exercises in this book underwent extensive testing at training programs around the world. For all of the pilot site leaders and trainees who volunteered to "test run" this work and provided critically important feedback throughout the method refinement and writing process, we cannot thank you enough. In particular, we are deeply grateful to the following supervisors and trainees who tested exercises and/or provided invaluable feedback:

- Ennio Ammendola, Ohio State University, Columbus, OH, United States
- Sara Bernardelli and Chris Kelly, private practice, Verona, Italy
- Kara L. Buda and Joseph Carter, City University of New York, New York, NY, United States
- David Disabato, Kent State University, Stow, OH, United States
- Maddi Gervasio and Annette Schieffelin, St. John's University, New York, NY, United States
- Jeffrey Goldman, private practice, New York, NY, United States
- Brooke Wachtler, private practice, New York, NY, United States

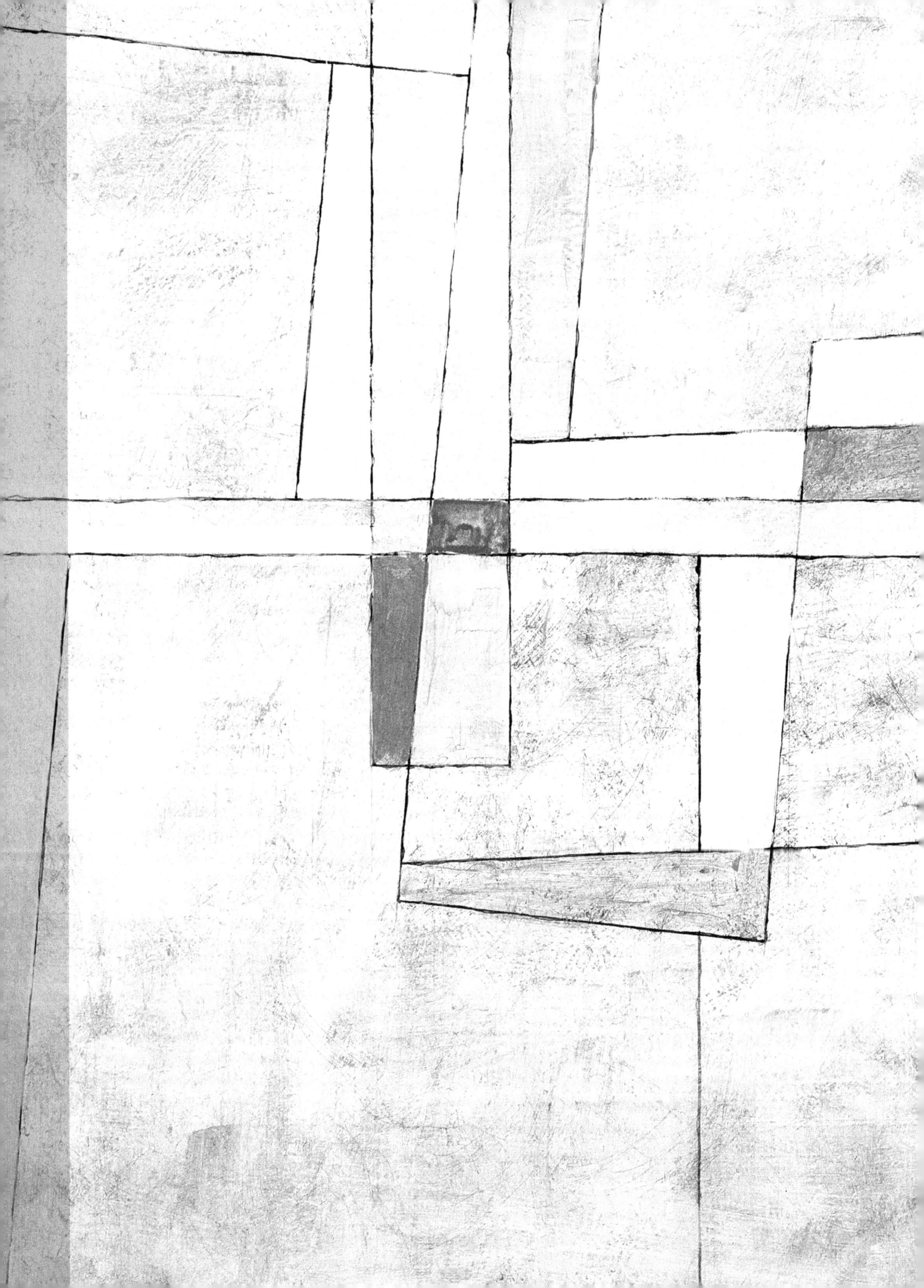

Overview and Instructions

In Part I, we provide an overview of deliberate practice, including how it can be integrated into clinical training programs for rational emotive behavior therapy (REBT), and instructions for performing the deliberate practice exercises in Part II. **We encourage both trainers and trainees to read both Chapters 1 and 2 before performing the deliberate practice exercises for the first time.**

Chapter 1 provides a foundation for the rest of the book by introducing important concepts related to deliberate practice and its role in psychotherapy training more broadly and REBT training more specifically. We also individually review the 12 skills from the exercises in Part II.

Chapter 2 lays out the basic, most essential instructions for performing the REBT deliberate practice exercises. They are designed to be quick and simple and provide you with just enough information to get started without being overwhelmed by too much information. Chapter 3 in Part III provides more in-depth guidance, which we encourage you to read once you are comfortable with the basic instructions in Chapter 2.

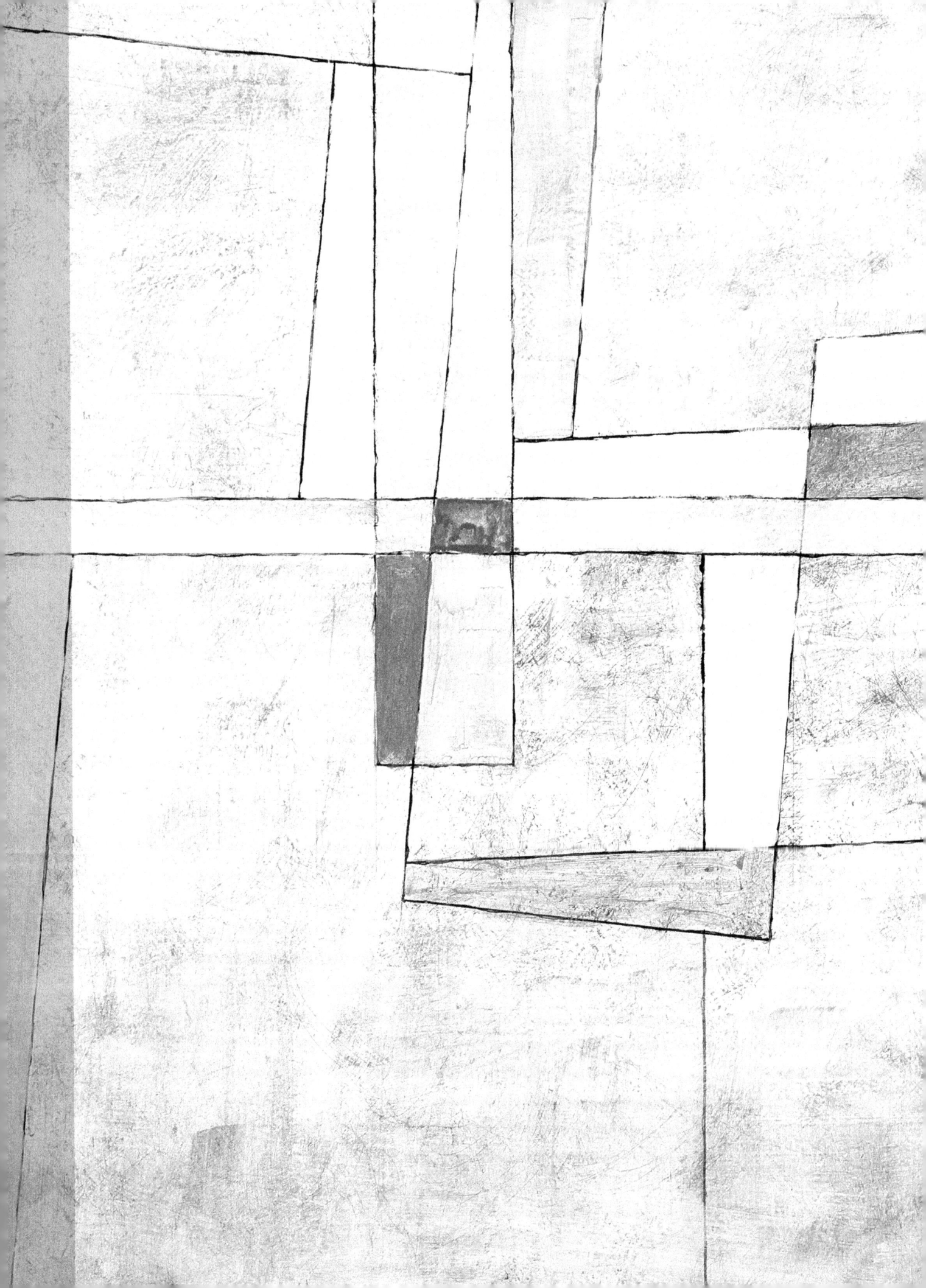

Introduction and Overview of Deliberate Practice and Rational Emotive Behavior Therapy

When training individuals in rational emotive behavior therapy (REBT), a common reaction from participants is that it sounds a lot like cognitive behavior therapy (CBT). As the pioneering form of CBT, there are many similarities but several unique differences. Another typical response from new trainees is that REBT is a simple approach to psychotherapy. Although some may agree that on the surface it appears simple, the application of REBT to real clients with a variety of clinical problems and emotional and behavioral disturbances is anything but easy. If that were the case, there would be no REBT practitioners because everyone would be solving their own problems. Listening to lectures on REBT or reading books on the theory can be very misleading. The intricacies of the theory become evident when trainees and practitioners begin to apply the skills. Upon review of Ray DiGiuseppe, Kristene Doyle, and Mark Terjesen's collective early experiences of REBT under the direct mentorship of its founder, Dr. Albert Ellis, it became clear that there were elements of deliberate practice embedded in our training and clinical practice, albeit not as structured or explicit. Albert Ellis required that we audio record our therapy sessions and play them during clinical supervision, and he would ask which aspects or skills in REBT were found to be more challenging in our practice, which is consistent with a deliberate practice approach to skill development. Dr. Ellis would not tell us what to do but would work with us to identify strategies to build our skills, and we would often practice these skills during group supervision. Suggestions were made about how to enhance our practice of REBT, such as being given a homework assignment between supervision sessions to listen to our session recordings and identify what we think we could have done better and practice what we could have said. Always a supportive supervisor, Al would follow up with us regarding our insights and provide reinforcement. Deliberate practice as it is presented in this series, and specifically in this book on REBT, is an organic next step or ingredient to the high-quality training we all received. The addition of continuing to work on one or several of the specific skills addressed in this book until a sense of mastery is achieved by the trainee as agreed on by an expert REBT supervisor serves to promote further professional development. The exercises provided for each of the skills included in this

https://doi.org/10.1037/0000334-001

Deliberate Practice in Rational Emotive Behavior Therapy, by M. D. Terjesen, K. A. Doyle, R. A. DiGiuseppe, A. Vaz, and T. Rousmaniere

book contain different clinical presentations of emotional and behavioral problems with varying levels of difficulty to allow the reader the opportunity to enhance their REBT skills as well as develop their own unique style of delivering REBT.

Overview of the Deliberate Practice Exercises

The main focus of the book is a series of 14 exercises that have been thoroughly tested and modified based on feedback from REBT trainers and trainees. Each of the first 12 exercises represents an essential REBT skill. The last two are more comprehensive, consisting of an annotated REBT transcript and improvised mock therapy sessions that teach practitioners how to integrate all these skills into more expansive clinical scenarios. Table 1.1 presents the 12 skills that are covered in these exercises.

Throughout the exercises, trainees work in pairs under the guidance of a supervisor and role-play as a client and a therapist, switching back and forth between the two roles. Each of the 12 skill-focused exercises consists of multiple scripted client statements grouped by difficulty—beginner, intermediate, and advanced—that calls for a specific skill. For each skill, trainees are asked to read through and absorb the description of the skill, its criteria, and some examples of it. The trainee playing the client then reads the statements. The trainee playing the therapist then responds in a way that demonstrates the appropriate skill. Trainee therapists will have the option of improvising and supplying their own response or, if they have trouble coming up with one, reading aloud an example response supplied in the exercise.

After each client statement and therapist response couplet is practiced several times, the trainees will stop to receive feedback from the supervisor. Guided by the supervisor, the trainees will be instructed to try statement–response couplets several times, working their way down the list. In consultation with the supervisor, trainees will go through the exercises, starting with the least challenging and moving through to more advanced levels. The triad (supervisor–client–therapist) will have the opportunity to discuss whether exercises present too much or too little challenge and adjust up or down depending on the assessment.

Trainees, in consultation with supervisors, can decide which skills they wish to practice and for how long. On the basis of our testing experience, we have found practice sessions

TABLE 1.1. The 12 Rational Emotive Behavior Therapy Skills Presented in the Deliberate Practice Exercises

Beginner Skills	Intermediate Skills	Advanced Skills
1. Psychoeducation about rational emotive behavior therapy's ABC model	5. Assessing irrational beliefs about the activating event	9. Empirical disputation of irrational beliefs
2. Psychoeducation about dysfunctional versus functional negative emotions and behaviors	6. Prioritizing which irrational beliefs to target for change	10. Semantic disputation of irrational beliefs
3. Agreement on the session goals	7. Teaching the belief–consequence connection	11. Constructing full rational alternative beliefs to replace irrational beliefs
4. Clarifying inferences from irrational beliefs	8. Functional disputation of irrational beliefs	12. Collaborative homework development

last about 1 to 1.25 hours to receive maximum benefit. After this, trainees become saturated and need a break.

Ideally, REBT learners will both gain confidence and achieve competence by practicing these exercises. *Competence* is defined here as the ability to perform an REBT skill in a manner that is flexible and responsive to the client. Skills have been chosen that are considered essential to REBT and that practitioners often find challenging to implement.

The skills identified in this book are not comprehensive in the sense of representing all one needs to learn to become a competent REBT clinician. Some skills will present particular challenges for trainees. A short history of REBT and a brief description of the deliberate practice methodology are provided to explain how we have arrived at the union between them.

The Goals of This Book

The primary goal of this book is to help trainees achieve competence in core REBT skills. Therefore, the expression of that skill or competency may look somewhat different across clients or even within a session with the same client.

The REBT deliberate practice exercises are designed to achieve the following:

1. Help REBT therapists develop the ability to apply the skills in a range of clinical situations.

2. Move the skills into procedural memory (Squire, 2004) so that REBT therapists can access them even when they are tired, stressed, overwhelmed, or discouraged.

3. Provide REBT therapists in training with an opportunity to exercise the particular skill using a style and language that is congruent with who they are.

4. Provide the opportunity to use the REBT skills in response to varying client statements and affect that represent a range of clinical problems. This is designed to build confidence to adopt skills in a broad range of circumstances within different client contexts.

5. Provide REBT therapists in training with many opportunities to fail and then correct their failed response on the basis of feedback. This helps build confidence and persistence.

Finally, this book aims to help trainees discover their own personal learning style so they can continue their professional development long after their formal training is concluded.

Who Can Benefit From This Book?

This book is designed to be used in multiple contexts, including in graduate-level courses, supervision, postgraduate training, and continuing education programs. It assumes the following:

1. The trainer is knowledgeable about and competent in REBT.

2. The trainer can provide good demonstrations of how to use REBT skills across a range of therapeutic situations via role-play. Or the trainer has access to examples of REBT being demonstrated through the many psychotherapy video examples available.

3. The trainer can provide feedback to students regarding how to craft or improve their application of REBT skills.

4. Trainees will have accompanying reading, such as books and articles, that explain the theory, research, and rationale of REBT and each particular skill. Recommended reading for each skill is provided in the sample syllabus (Appendix C).

The exercises covered in this book were piloted in seven training sites from two continents (North America and Europe). This book is designed for trainers and trainees from different cultural backgrounds worldwide.

This book is also designed for those who are training at all career stages, from beginning trainees, including those who have never worked with real clients, to seasoned therapists. All exercises feature guidance for assessing the adjusting the difficulty to precisely target the needs of each individual learner. The term *trainee* in this book is used broadly, referring to anyone in the field of professional mental health who endeavors to acquire REBT psychotherapy skills. For further guidance on how to improve multicultural deliberate practice skills, see the forthcoming book *Deliberate Practice in Multicultural Therapy* (Harris et al., in press).

Deliberate Practice in Psychotherapy Training

How does one become an expert in their professional field? What is trainable, and what is simply beyond our reach due to innate or uncontrollable factors? Questions such as these touch on our fascination with expert performers and their development. A mixture of awe, admiration, and even confusion surrounds people such as Mozart, Leonardo da Vinci, or more contemporary top performers, such as basketball legend Michael Jordan and chess virtuoso Garry Kasparov. What accounts for their consistently superior professional results? Evidence suggests that the amount of or time spent on a particular type of training is a key factor in developing expertise in virtually all domains (Ericsson & Pool, 2016). Deliberate practice is an evidence-based method that can improve performance in an effective and reliable manner.

The concept of deliberate practice has its origins in a classic study by K. Anders Ericsson and colleagues (1993). They found that the amount of time practicing a skill and the quality of the time spent doing so were key factors predicting mastery and acquisition. They identified five key activities in learning and mastering skills: (a) observing one's own work, (b) getting expert feedback, (c) setting small incremental learning goals just beyond the performer's ability, (d) engaging in repetitive behavioral rehearsal of specific skills, and (e) continuously assessing performance. Ericsson and his colleagues termed this process *deliberate practice*, a cyclical process that is illustrated in Figure 1.1.

Research has shown that lengthy engagement in deliberate practice is associated with expert performance across a variety of professional fields, such as medicine, sports, music, chess, computer programming, and mathematics (Ericsson et al., 2018). People may associate deliberate practice with the widely known "10,000-hour rule" popularized by Malcolm Gladwell in his 2008 book, *Outliers*, although the actual number of hours required for expertise varies by field and by individual (Ericsson & Pool, 2016). This idea, though, perpetuates two misunderstandings. First, that this is the number of deliberate practice hours that everyone needs to attain expertise, no matter the domain. In fact, there can be considerable variability in how many hours are required.

FIGURE 1.1. Cycle of Deliberate Practice

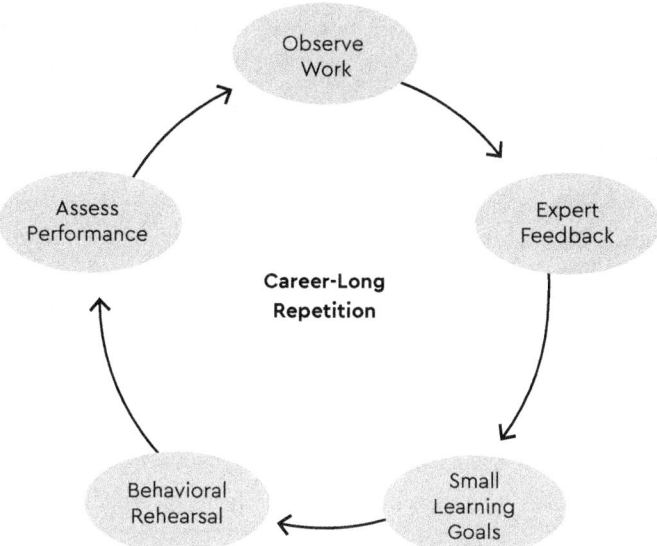

Note. From *Deliberate Practice in Emotion-Focused Therapy* (p. 7), by R. N. Goldman, A. Vaz, and T. Rousmaniere, 2021, American Psychological Association (https://doi.org/10.1037/0000227–000). Copyright 2021 by the American Psychological Association.

The second misunderstanding is that engagement in 10,000 hours of work performance will lead one to become an expert in that domain. This misunderstanding holds considerable significance for the field of psychotherapy, where hours of work experience with clients has traditionally been used as a measure of proficiency (Rousmaniere, 2016). Research suggests that the amount of experience alone does not predict therapist effectiveness (Goldberg, Babins-Wagner, et al., 2016; Goldberg, Rousmaniere, et al., 2016). It may be that the quality of deliberate practice is a key factor.

Psychotherapy scholars, recognizing the value of deliberate practice in other fields, have recently called for deliberate practice to be incorporated into training for mental health professionals (e.g., Bailey & Ogles, 2019; Hill et al., 2020; Rousmaniere et al., 2017; Taylor & Neimeyer, 2017; Tracey et al., 2015). There are, however, good reasons to question analogies made between psychotherapy and other professional fields, like sports or music, because by comparison psychotherapy is so complex and free-form. Sports have clearly defined goals, and classical music follows a written score. In contrast, the goals of psychotherapy shift with the unique presentation of each client at each session. Therapists do not have the luxury of following a score.

Instead, good psychotherapy is more like improvisational jazz (Noa Kageyama, as cited in Rousmaniere, 2016). In jazz improvisations, band members coconstruct a complex mixture of group collaboration, creativity, and interaction. Like psychotherapy, no two jazz improvisations are identical. However, improvisations are not a random collection of notes. They are grounded in a comprehensive theoretical understanding and technical proficiency that is only developed through continuous deliberate practice. For example, prominent jazz instructor Jerry Coker (1990) listed 18 skill areas that students must master, each of which has multiple discrete skills, including tone quality, intervals, chord arpeggios, scales, patterns, and licks. In this sense, more creative and artful improvisations are actually a reflection of a previous commitment to repetitive skill practice and acquisition. As legendary jazz musician Miles Davis put it, "You have to play a long time to be able to play like yourself" (Cook, 2005, p. 34).

The main idea that we would like to stress here is that we want deliberate practice to help REBT therapists become themselves. The idea is to learn the skills so that you have them on hand when you want them. Practice the skills to make them your own. Incorporate those aspects that feel right for you. Ongoing and effortful deliberate practice should not be an impediment to flexibility and creativity. As in the arts, deliberate practice should enhance flexibility and creativity. We recognize and celebrate that psychotherapy is an ever-shifting encounter and by no means want it to become or feel formulaic. Strong REBT therapists mix an eloquent integration of previously acquired skills with properly attuned flexibility. The core REBT responses provided are meant as templates or possibilities, rather than "answers." Please interpret and apply them as you see fit, in a way that makes sense to you. We encourage flexible and improvisational play!

Simulation-Based Mastery Learning

Deliberate practice uses simulation-based mastery learning exercises (Ericsson, 2004; McGaghie et al., 2014). That is, the stimulus material for training consists of "contrived social situations that mimic problems, events, or conditions that arise in professional encounters" (McGaghie et al., 2014, p. 375). A key component of this approach is that the stimuli being used in training are sufficiently similar to the real-world experiences, so that what they mimic provokes similar reactions. This facilitates *state-dependent learning*, where professionals acquire skills in the same psychological environment where they will have to perform the skills (Fisher & Craik, 1977). For example, pilots train with flight simulators that present mechanical failures and dangerous weather conditions, and surgeons practice with surgical simulators that present medical complications. Training in simulations with challenging stimuli increases professionals' capacity to perform effectively under stress. For the psychotherapy training exercises in this book, the "simulators" are typical client statements that might actually be presented in the course of therapy sessions and call upon the use of the particular skill.

Declarative Versus Procedural Knowledge

Declarative knowledge is what a person can understand, write, or speak about. It often refers to factual information that can be consciously recalled through memory and often can be acquired relatively quickly. In contrast, procedural learning is implicit in memory, and "usually requires *repetition of an activity*, and associated learning is demonstrated through *improved task performance*" (Koziol & Budding, 2012, pp. 2694, emphasis added). *Procedural knowledge* is what a person can perform, especially under stress (Squire, 2004). People can display a wide difference between their declarative and procedural knowledge. For example, an "armchair quarterback" is a person who understands and talks about athletics well but would have trouble performing those skills at a professional ability level. Likewise, most dance, music, or theatre critics have a very high ability to write about their subjects but would be flummoxed if asked to perform them.

The sweet spot for deliberate practice is the gap between declarative and procedural knowledge. In other words, effortful practice should target those skills that the trainee could write a good paper about but would have trouble actually performing with a real client. We start with declarative knowledge, learning skills theoretically and observing others perform them. Once learned, with the help of deliberate practice, we work toward the development of procedural learning, with the aim of therapists having "automatic" access to each of the skills that they can pull on when necessary.

Let us turn to a little theoretical background on REBT to help contextualize the skills of the book and how they fit into the greater training model.

REBT: Theoretical Overview

REBT is an evidence-based psychotherapy originally designed by Albert Ellis (1957, 1962, 1994) to treat anxiety and relationship problems, but which grew into a transdiagnostic approach used to treat a wide range of emotional and behavioral problems. REBT grew out of Ellis's attempt to use principles of Stoic and other philosophical approaches to control one's emotional and behavioral symptoms. REBT was one of the first approaches to psychotherapy to advocate the empirical, scientific testing of therapy outcome. It also believes that people are psychologically adjusted when they use the scientific method to analyze their own thinking. As such, REBT was one of the first modern approaches to CBT (D. David et al., 2018).

REBT maintains that people's beliefs are the principal factors that trigger their emotional and behavioral symptoms. REBT maintains that irrational beliefs, which are rigid, illogical, antiempirical, and block our goals, lead to unhealthy, disturbed negative emotions and maladaptive behaviors. Correspondingly, rational beliefs, which are flexible, logical, consistent with reality, and helpful in reaching goals, lead to adaptive, nondisturbed negative emotions and adaptive behaviors. Irrational and rational beliefs are imperative or evaluative thoughts. That is, they might lead individuals to be demanding of themselves, others, or the situation or to evaluate the situation in an unhealthy way by thinking it to be awful, too difficult to deal with, or attach a rating of worth to oneself, others, or life conditions.

Irrational beliefs do not represent the person's perceptions about a negative distortion or the perception of reality, but how the person evaluates their perceptions of reality and what they think reality should be. Therefore, clinical interventions based on REBT focus on identifying and examining and challenging a client's irrational beliefs and replacing them with more rational beliefs. REBT represents a philosophical approach to therapy because it focuses on these evaluative and imperative beliefs and not the presence or absence of negative distortions of reality.

REBT highlights several beliefs as more central to disturbance than others are. The first is the idea of demandingness. Demandingness represents an unrealistic and absolute expectation that events or individuals will be the way a person desires them to be—that is, "Because I want it a certain way, it should be that way." Most other irrational beliefs are thought to be a derivative of this process and are discussed later. The rational alternative to demandingness is acceptance. Acceptance represents the acknowledgment that one prefers the world, themselves, or people to be a certain way but that the world is as it is. Acceptance of a reality that is different from how you want it to be is the first step to coping with problems.

Research (DiGiuseppe et al., 2020) has demonstrated that a second irrational belief (global evaluation of human worth) appears to stand on its own and is an independent belief construct from other irrational beliefs. Global evaluations of human worth, either of the self or others, imply that human beings can be rated and that some people are worthless, or at least less valuable than others are. People often base their ratings of worth based on specific behaviors. The rational alternative to this idea is that all humans have equal value and are important regardless of behavior; however, individuals are still responsible for their behaviors. Negative global evaluations of the self can lead to depression, shame, guilt, or anxiety, while negative global evaluations of others can lead to anger, contempt, and hatred. REBT stresses that people strive to achieve unconditional self-acceptance rather than self-esteem. We accept ourselves (and others) with our flaws and failures and recognize that we have worth despite them.

Another central irrational belief is that of frustration or discomfort intolerance. This idea represents a demand for comfort and a belief in one's inability to survive or tolerate discomfort and frustration. The rational alternative to this idea is that, even when things might be difficult, one can be strong and live with discomfort to accomplish long-term goals.

The fourth of the core irrational beliefs is the idea of awfulizing. This occurs when a person believes that an event is 100%+ bad or worse, that nothing could be worse, that nothing good can come from this, and that they cannot overcome this (Dryden, 2020). The rational alternative to this idea is that although bad things may happen, and we will validate and acknowledge that clinically, we do not attach the label or belief that this bad event is truly awful or beyond bad.

REBT takes a strong theoretical stance on human emotions that is different from other clinical approaches. First, REBT maintains that for each negative human emotion, people have several possible alternative emotions that they can experience along a continuum of intensity. Some of these negative emotions are unhealthy and disturbed and prevent us from achieving our goals. Other emotions are healthy and adaptive yet negative in that they motivate us to recognize problems and work toward a resolution. Adverse activating events will always occur in life. Our emotional and behavioral reactions to such events are determined by our beliefs about the adverse events. The theory and science of REBT proposes that irrational beliefs lead to the unhealthy disturbed negative emotions and rational beliefs lead to the healthy, adaptive negative emotions, not neutral feelings. Thus, tolerance of negative events and negative emotions is important to achieving psychological adjustment. In REBT, psychological adjustment comes from acceptance of the world, of ourselves and others, and of our frustrations and discomforts.

The identification, challenging, and replacement of irrational beliefs are the most common therapeutic activities in REBT. Teaching clients to practice this set of verbal skills remains the most frequent task used in clinical work. However, from its inception (A. Ellis, 1957), REBT has advocated the use of a wide range of emotive, imaginal, and behavioral activities to facilitate change. It was one of the first approaches to advocate between-session homework activities, which is addressed in Exercise 12. This remains a crucial part of the therapy. Helping clients use these varied tasks to think, feel, and act differently between sessions is a crucial set of skills in REBT.

The exercises included in this book are aimed at developing REBT skills across all the concepts mentioned previously (see also the later section describing the skills that are covered in this book's exercises).

The Role of Deliberate Practice in REBT Training

Training in REBT—like deliberate practice more broadly—has always made the distinction between declarative and procedural knowledge. In fact, like the discussion of deliberate practice in general, we have for decades made the analogy between learning REBT and learning an athletic skill. Knowing the REBT theory and what to do in REBT does not mean that you can or will do it. Practicing the skills is crucial. For the 47 years that the most senior coauthor of this book (R.A.D.) has been involved in teaching REBT, the Albert Ellis Institute has included training activities similar to, but not using the term, of deliberate practice.

The Albert Ellis Institute has been offering a primary certificate training program in REBT for more than 50 years and has conservatively trained 25,000 clinicians in REBT around the world. This training has always involved three types of activities. First, they learn declarative knowledge about the theory and activities of REBT from readings and lectures. Second, a senior REBT trainer provides a demonstration of a therapy session. The therapists are cognizant of clearly demonstrating specific skills to provide modelling of the skills for the learners. Finally, the participants pair up and do what we have called peer counseling. The first person takes the role of the client and presents a minor emotional or behavioral problem to the second trainee who plays the therapist with the objective being that they demonstrate the REBT skills learned. The therapist then receives feedback on their performance. Then the two participants change roles. Over the course of the training, the expectations of demonstration of REBT skills increases building off the prior demonstration and feedback. Over the years, we have had numerous discussions concerning how to identify the skills, the order of skill difficulty, and the sequence in which the skills would be taught. REBT has always included deliberate practice skill training in therapist training, just not as explicitly as done within this book. In the supervisory training practicum offered at the Albert Ellis Institute, we have long advocated the importance of supervisors teaching the declarative knowledge concerning what the therapist would do, then modelling exactly what the therapist would say, emphasizing the tone of voice, and then having the therapist actually do it. Next, the supervisor asks the therapist to demonstrate the response with an actual client (Doyle et al., 2022).

Originally, we had trainees make audio recordings of their peer counseling skills and then met to review the recordings and provide feedback. However, all the trainees usually made the same mistakes, and we would listen to the same error over again on each trainee's recordings. We corrected this process and reduced the length of our training to achieve competency in the basic REBT skills mentioned here by providing trainees with immediate feedback after live versus recorded practice sessions. So immediate feedback of one skill at a time appears to be the best way to proceed and is consistent with the deliberate practice approach toward developing clinical skills.

Once trainees have mastered the skills, it can still be difficult for them to produce the skills in a sequential order, as they have to do in an actual therapy session. This book does not follow the reader's course of development to that level, but this is what we hope to teach in Exercises 13 and 14. So we advise you to expect that you will need more trials to learn to put these skills together into a coherent therapy session.

We want to also recognize that we focus here on REBT skills. REBT skills build on the common factors in psychotherapy, especially the therapist skills of expressing empathy, congruence, and achieving a good therapeutic alliance, which are the cornerstones of good clinical practice and advocated by all REBT trainers (DiGiuseppe, 2022).

The deliberate practice exercises in this book are not sufficient by themselves for obtaining full competence in REBT. However, they closely represent the criteria set by the International Training Standards Committee on REBT as the necessary skills to achieve the primary certificate in REBT from the Albert Ellis Institute. The skills included here are suited to a first course in REBT and are presented in a sample syllabus (see Appendix C). Trainees should have more extensive exposure to REBT theory and application in coursework and readings. We look forward to developing more deliberate practice exercises that will include more advanced level skills.

REBT Skills in Deliberate Practice

The REBT Skills Presented in Exercises 1 Through 12

When clients present clinical problems to a therapist, they usually start by identifying a strong disturbed emotion or an activating event that troubles them. That is, they present with either the A (activating event) or the C (emotional and/or behavioral consequence) in the ABC model. The skill exercises presented in this book follow the format that represents how the therapist would progress through helping a client go through the steps of doing an REBT analysis for such a problem. The skills are presented in the sequence that therapists usually follow in applying REBT to a clinical problem. The beginning steps represent teaching the client about REBT, the ABC model, and how therapists identify the A and C and then the Bs (beliefs). Also presented are the steps in achieving agreement on the goals and tasks of therapy, which form two steps in the formation of the therapeutic alliance and are necessary to move forward to the more advanced steps of disputing the irrational beliefs, developing rational alternative beliefs, and collaborating on homework. As it turns out, this order of presentation also represents the order of difficulty that trainees have reported to us over the years. These 12 skills go from a beginning level early in the REBT sequence, to later skills that are of more moderate difficulty, then to the late-stage skills that are more advanced and more difficult. The order of the skills appears in Table 1.1. We want to emphasize that the skills presented here help therapists to both build a collaborative therapeutic alliance and provide information to construct a case conceptualization.

The beginner-level exercises consist of the most basic REBT skills used in most sessions. This includes teaching clients about the ABC model (Exercise 1). This skill provides clients with an orientation to think about whether their problem is an activating event, their beliefs and thoughts, or the emotions and behaviors they have. Understanding these distinctions will make it easier for clients to identify the goals of therapy and the tasks that will be used to achieve them. The second skill involves psychoeducation about the difference between various types of emotions and behaviors (Exercise 2). We believe that learning these distinctions will also help clarify the goals of the therapy with the client. This leads to the next skill, which is getting explicit agreement on the goals of therapy (Exercise 3). The final beginner skill (Exercise 4) involves clarifying the differences between inferences or cognitive distortions as opposed to irrational beliefs. Understanding this distinction helps the client focus on the main core activities of REBT and also helps the therapist and client establish agreement on the tasks of therapy.

The intermediate skills involve identifying the core aspects of the ABC model and beginning the process of change. Exercise 5 involves the therapist and client collaborating on assessing which irrational belief(s) the client has about the problematic activating event that leads them to experience unhealthy negative emotions or behaviors. Clients usually endorse more than one irrational belief, and in Exercise 6, the therapist helps the client prioritize which belief they want to change first. Again, this skill is crucial in establishing the agreement on the task aspect of the therapeutic alliance. Once we identify the client's irrational beliefs, a mistake that we have found that beginning REBT clinicians often make is that they either simply try to replace the belief or to dispute it. Although an important part of the REBT process, challenging or replacing irrational beliefs makes no sense unless the client understands the relationship of the beliefs to their emotions and behaviors. This is the focus of Exercise 7, and, again, this skill helps foster agreement on the task aspect of the therapeutic alliance. Once the therapist proceeds through these skills, it is time to get to the process of changing the irrational beliefs. This begins in Exercise 8, where therapists learn the easiest of the disputation strategies: functional disputation of irrational beliefs.

The advanced level skills involve two more difficult disputation strategies: the empirical disputation of irrational beliefs (Exercise 9) and the semantic disputation of irrational beliefs (Exercise 10). In the next step, the therapist helps the client construct a new alternative rational replacement belief (Exercise 11). Once this is done, therapists will engage in the most difficult task covered here, which is collaboratively developing homework activities for the client to do between sessions (Exercise 12).

Overview of the Book's Structure

This book is organized into three parts. Part I contains this chapter and Chapter 2, which provides basic instructions on how to perform these exercises. We found through testing that providing too many instructions up-front overwhelmed trainers and trainees, and as a result, they skipped past them. Therefore, we kept these instructions as brief and simple as possible to focus only on the most essential information that trainers and trainees will need to get started with the exercises. Further guidelines for getting the most from deliberate practice are provided in Chapter 3, and additional instructions for monitoring and adjusting the difficulty of the exercises are provided in Appendix A. **Do not skip the instructions in Chapter 2, and be sure to read the additional guidelines and instructions in Chapter 3 and Appendix A once you are comfortable with the basic instructions.**

Part II contains the 12 skill-focused exercises, which are ordered as they would be used in an actual therapy situation. This order also corresponds to the difficulty level of the skills: beginner, intermediate, and advanced (see Table 1.1). The discussion of each of the 12 skills contain a brief overview of the exercise, a list of criteria for mastering the relevant skill, example client–therapist interactions to help guide trainees, and step-by-step instructions for conducting that exercise. The client statements and sample therapist responses are then presented, also organized by difficulty (beginner, intermediate, and advanced). The statements and responses are presented separately so that the trainee playing the therapist has more freedom to improvise responses without being influenced by the sample responses, which the trainee should turn to only if they have difficulty improvising their own responses.

While the focus of each scripted response was written explicitly for that specific skill exercise, we took considerable effort in crafting prompts and responses that provide an opportunity for the clinician to see the application of REBT skills. We consistently presented client prompts for five key emotional experiences (anger, depression, guilt, anxiety, and jealousy). Although the prompts differed in background, context, and presenting problem, having these key emotions appear consistently allows for readers to consider all 12 skills across these five key emotions. That is, readers will become more skilled in applying REBT across these different emotions because these are the ones that we believe they are most likely to experience in clinical practice. As they become more proficient in the application of these skills for treatment of these emotions, it is expected that they can generalize these REBT skills to other emotional and behavioral consequences.

Another important distinguishing feature of the client prompts across the 12 exercises is the inclusion of consequences that are both emotional and behavioral in nature to allow for readers to develop skills in working with both types of problems. At the core of REBT is cognitive restructuring or disputation, and, for the three disputation exercises, we kept the client prompts identical. This allows trainees to see how best to dispute these irrational beliefs across three types of disputation strategies. Relatedly, we made efforts to balance the specific client irrational beliefs to provide the reader with more opportunities to practice the different disputation skills for different types of irrational beliefs presented by clients. That is, in Exercises 8 through 10 all client prompts are the same, but the disputation skill and criteria vary across the skills.

In developing these skills and the practice scenarios, we put considerable thought into how to help clinicians develop these specific REBT skills through deliberate practice in a way that also considers the process of REBT as a therapeutic approach. Given that each prompt does not provide an opportunity for a back-and-forth dialogue with a client, there were times when we considered what else may be important clinically but perhaps not be as specific to this skill. That is, when you read a prompt for a specific skill, you may be tempted to think that you would do something else first before demonstrating this skill. As an example, you may think it important to develop goals in a session before disputing. And you would be correct within a natural therapeutic context. We ordered the skills to reflect what may happen within a typical REBT session. That is, psychoeducation about REBT (Exercise 1) would come before functional disputation (Exercise 8). We encourage you to focus on the specific skills for each specific skill set and assume that the clinician and client have already done the prior steps competently. Do not be tempted, as an example, to provide psychoeducation (Exercise 1) when trying to demonstrate the skills of functional disputation (Exercise 8). We simply highlight this for additional context when comparing one's improvised response with the scripted therapist response.

The last two exercises in Part II provide opportunities to practice the 12 skills within simulated psychotherapy sessions. Exercise 13 provides a sample psychotherapy session transcript in which the REBT skills are used and clearly labelled, thereby demonstrating how they might flow together in an actual therapy session. REBT trainees are invited to run through the sample transcript with one playing the therapist and the other playing the client to get a feel for how a session might unfold. Exercise 14 provides suggestions for undertaking mock sessions, as well as client profiles ordered by difficulty (beginner, intermediate, and advanced) that trainees can use for improvised role-plays.

Part III contains Chapter 3, which provides additional guidance for trainers and trainees. While Chapter 2 is more procedural, Chapter 3 covers big-picture issues. It highlights six key points for getting the most out of deliberate practice and describes the importance of appropriate responsiveness, attending to trainee well-being and respecting their privacy, and trainer self-evaluation, among other topics.

Three appendixes conclude this book. Appendix A provides instructions for monitoring and adjusting the difficulty of each exercise as needed. It provides a Deliberate Practice Reaction Form for the trainee playing the therapist to complete to indicate whether the exercise is too easy or too difficult. Appendix B includes a Deliberate Practice Diary Form that can be used to during a training session's final evaluation to process trainees' experiences, but its primary purpose is to provide trainees a format to explore and record their experiences while engaging in additional, between-session deliberate practice activities without the supervisor. Appendix C presents a sample syllabus demonstrating how the 14 deliberate practice exercises and other support material can be integrated into a wider REBT training course. Instructors can choose to modify the syllabus or pick elements of it to integrate into their own courses.

Downloadable versions of this book's appendixes, including a color version of the Deliberate Practice Reaction Form, can be found in the "Clinician and Practitioner Resources" tab online (https://www.apa.org/pubs/books/deliberate-practice-rational-emotive-behavior-therapy).

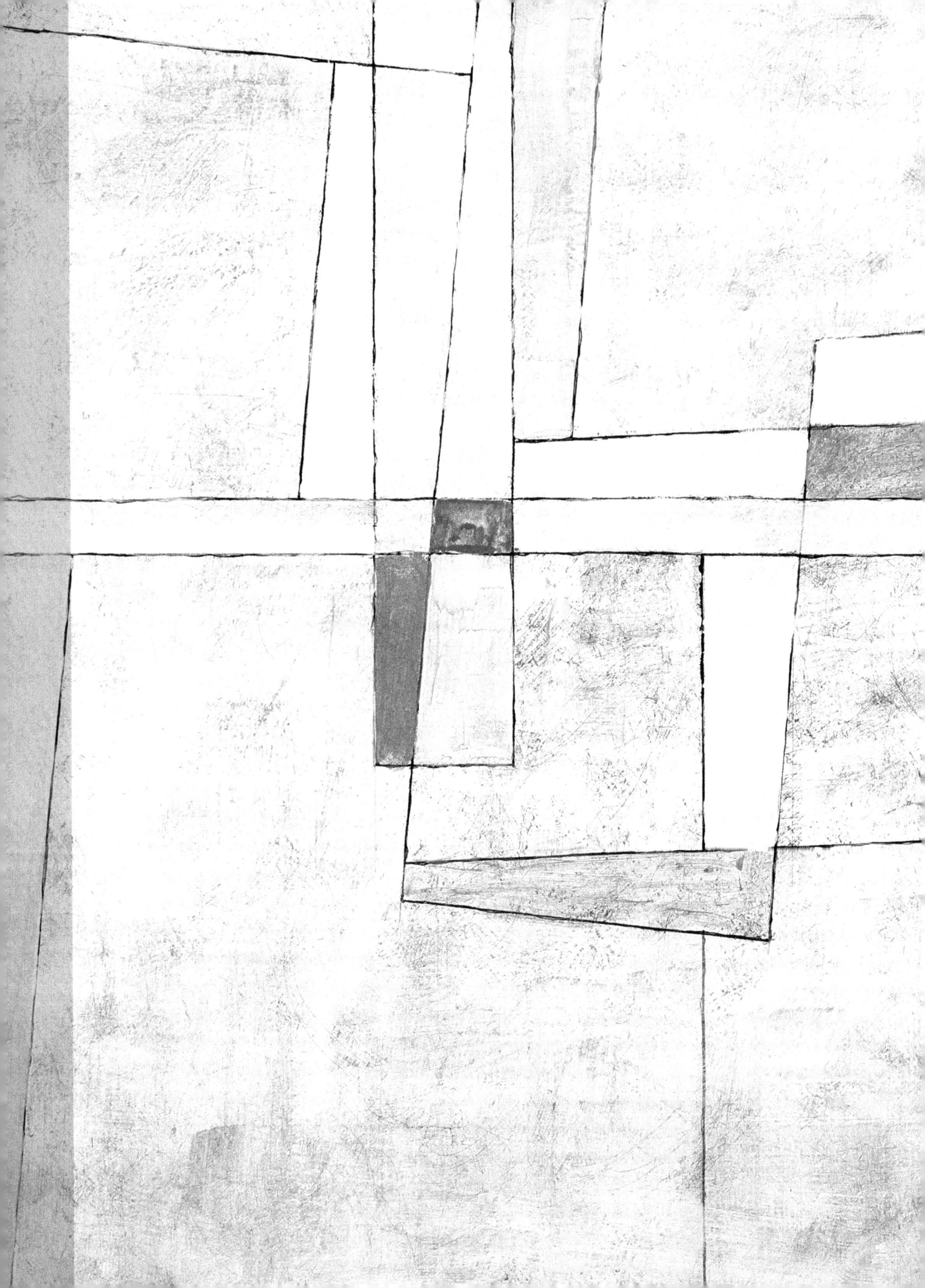

Instructions for the Rational Emotive Behavior Therapy Deliberate Practice Exercises

This chapter provides basic instructions that are common to all the exercises in this book. More specific instructions are provided in each exercise. Chapter 3 also provides important guidance for trainees and trainers that will help them get the most out of deliberate practice. Appendix A offers additional instructions for monitoring and adjusting the difficulty of the exercises as needed after getting through all then client statements in a single difficulty level, including a Deliberate Practice Reaction Form the trainee playing the therapist can complete to indicate whether they found the statements too easy or too difficult. **Difficulty assessment is an important part of the deliberate practice process and should not be skipped.**

Overview

The deliberate practice exercises in this book involve role-plays of hypothetical situations in therapy. The role-play involves three people: one trainee role-plays the therapist, another trainee role-plays the client, and a trainer (professor/supervisor) observes and provides feedback. Alternatively, a peer can observe and provide feedback.

This book provides a script for each role-play, each with a client statement and also with an example therapist response. The client statements are graded in difficulty from beginning to advanced, although these difficulty grades are only estimates. The actual perceived difficulty of client statements is very subjective and varies widely by trainee. For example, some trainees may experience a stimulus of a client being angry as being easy to respond to, whereas another trainee may experience it as very difficult. Thus, it is important for trainees to provide difficulty assessments and adjustments to ensure that they are practicing at the right difficulty level: neither too easy nor too hard.

https://doi.org/10.1037/0000334-002

Deliberate Practice in Rational Emotive Behavior Therapy, by M. D. Terjesen, K. A. Doyle, R. A. DiGiuseppe, A. Vaz, and T. Rousmaniere

Time Frame

We recommend a 90-minute time block for every exercise, structured roughly as follows:

- First 20 minutes: Orientation. The trainer explains the rational emotive behavior therapy (REBT) skill and demonstrates the exercise procedure with a volunteer trainee.

- Middle 50 minutes: Trainees perform the exercise in pairs. The trainer or a peer provides feedback throughout this process and monitors and adjusts the exercise's difficulty as needed after each set of statements (see Appendix A for more information about difficulty assessment).

- Final 20 minutes: Review, feedback, and discussion.

Preparation

1. Every trainee will need their own copy of this book.

2. Each exercise requires the trainer to fill out a Deliberate Practice Reaction Form after completing all the statements from a single difficulty level. This form is available in the "Clinician and Practitioner Resources" tab online (https://www.apa.org/pubs/books/deliberate-practice-rational-emotive-behavior-therapy) and in Appendix A.

3. Trainees are grouped into pairs. One volunteers to role-play the therapist and one to role-play the client (they will switch roles after 15 minutes of practice). As noted previously, an observer who might be either the trainer or a fellow trainee will work with each pair.

The Role of the Trainer

The primary responsibilities of the trainer are as follows:

1. To provide corrective feedback, which includes both information about how well the trainees' response met expected criteria and any necessary guidance about how to improve the response.

2. To remind trainees to do difficulty assessments and adjustments after each level of client statements is completed (beginning, intermediate, and advanced).

How to Practice

Each exercise includes its own step-by-step instructions. Trainees should follow these instructions carefully because every step is important.

Skill Criteria

Each of the first 12 exercises focuses on one essential REBT skill with two to four skill criteria that describe the important components or principles for that skill.

The goal of the role-play is for trainees to practice improvising responses to the client statement in a manner that (a) is attuned to the client, (b) meets skill criteria as much

as possible, and (c) feels authentic for the trainee. Trainees are provided scripts with example therapist responses to give them a sense of how to incorporate the skill criteria into a response. **It is important, however, that trainees do not read the example responses verbatim in the role-plays!** Therapy is highly personal and improvisational; the goal of deliberate practice is to develop trainees' ability to improvise within a consistent framework. Memorizing scripted responses would be counterproductive for helping trainees learn to perform therapy that is responsive, authentic, and attuned to each individual client.

The example scripted responses were collaboratively designed with the aim to stay genuine to good therapy practice while also demonstrating the specific REBT skill. However, trainees' personal styles of therapy may differ slightly or greatly from that in the example scripts. It is essential that, over time, trainees develop their own style and voice, while simultaneously being able to intervene according to the model's principles and strategies. To facilitate this, the exercises in this book were designed to maximize opportunities for improvisational responses informed by the skill criteria and ongoing feedback. Trainees will note that some of the scripted responses do not meet all the skill criteria: These responses are provided as examples of flexible application of REBT skills in a manner that prioritizes attunement with the client.

The goal for the role-plays is for trainees to practice improvising responses to the client statements in a manner that

- is attuned to the client,
- meets as many of the skill criteria as possible, and
- feels authentic for the trainee.

Review, Feedback, and Discussion

The review and feedback sequence after each role-play has these two elements:

- First, the trainee who played the client **briefly** shares how it felt to be on the receiving end of the therapist's response. This can help assess how well trainees are attuning with the client.

- Second, the trainer provides **brief** feedback (less than 1 minute) based on the skill criteria for each exercise. Keep feedback specific, behavioral, and succinct to preserve time for skill rehearsal. If one trainer is teaching multiple pairs of trainees, the trainer walks around the room, observing the pairs and offering brief feedback. When the trainer is not available, the trainee playing the client gives peer feedback to the therapist, based on the skill criteria and how it felt to be on the receiving end of the intervention. Alternatively, a third trainee can observe and provide feedback.

Trainers (or peers) should remember to keep all feedback specific and brief and not to veer into discussions of theory. There are many other settings for extended discussion of REBT theory and research. In deliberate practice, it is of utmost importance to maximize time for continuous behavioral rehearsal via role-plays.

Final Evaluation

After both trainees have role-played the client and the therapist, the trainer provides an evaluation. Participants should engage in a short group discussion based on this evaluation. This discussion can provide ideas for where to focus homework and future deliberate practice sessions. To this end, Appendix B presents a Deliberate Practice Diary Form, which can also be downloaded from the "Clinician and Practitioner Resources" tab online (https://www.apa.org/pubs/books/deliberate-practice-rational-emotive-behavior-therapy). This form can be used as part of the final evaluation to help trainees process their experiences from that session with the supervisor. However, it is designed primarily to be used by trainees as a template for exploring and recording their thoughts and experiences between sessions, particularly when pursuing additional deliberate practice activities without the supervisor, such as rehearsing responses alone or if two or more trainees want to practice the exercises together—perhaps with another trainee filling the supervisor's role. Then, if they want, the trainees can discuss these experiences with the supervisor at the beginning of the next training session.

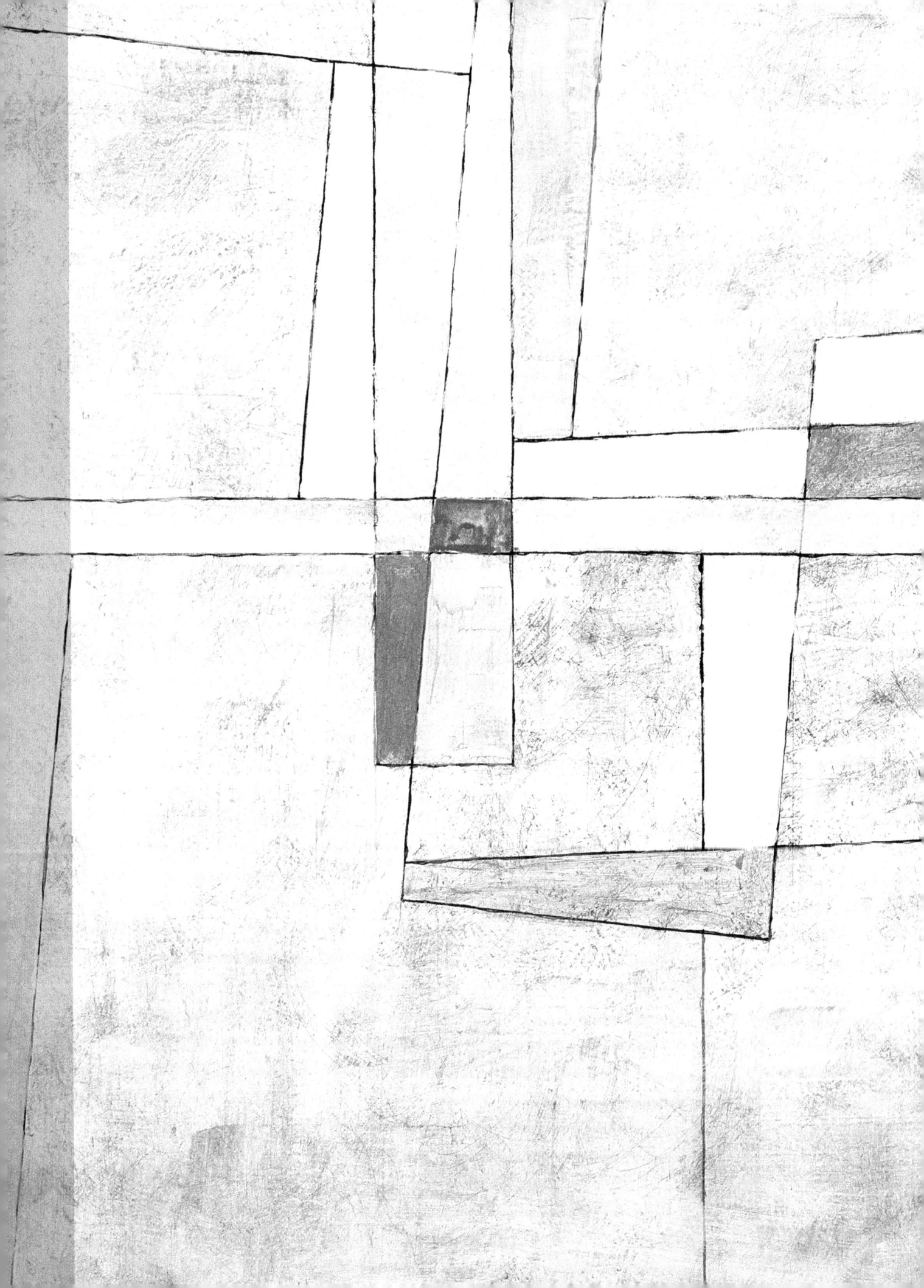

Deliberate Practice Exercises for Rational Emotive Behavior Therapy Skills

This section of the book provides 12 deliberate practice exercises for essential rational emotive behavior therapy (REBT) skills. These exercises are organized in a developmental sequence, from those that are more appropriate to someone just beginning REBT training to those who have progressed to a more advanced level. Although we anticipate that most trainers would use these exercises in the order we have suggested, some trainers may find it more appropriate to their training circumstances to use a different order. We also provide two comprehensive exercises that bring together the REBT skills using an annotated REBT session transcript and mock REBT sessions.

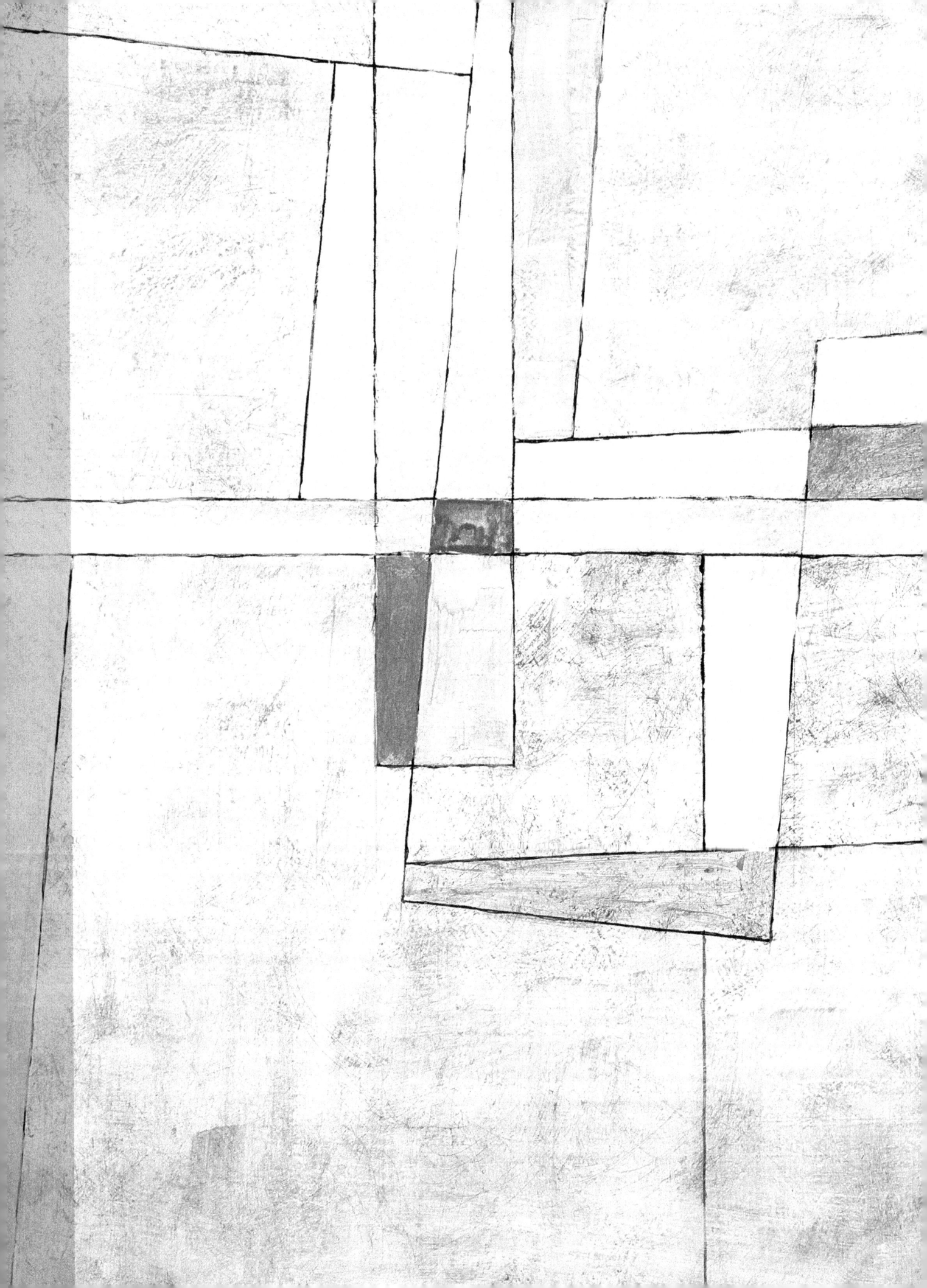

Psychoeducation About Rational Emotive Behavior Therapy's ABC Model

Preparations for Exercise 1

1. Read the instructions in Chapter 2.

2. Download the Deliberate Practice Reaction Form and the Deliberate Practice Diary Form at https://www.apa.org/pubs/books/deliberate-practice-rational-emotive-behavior-therapy (see the "Clinician and Practitioner Resources" tab; also available in Appendixes A and B, respectively).

Skill Description

Skill Difficulty Level: Beginner

Often, clients think that it is people or situations that cause their emotional distress or behavioral difficulties. Rational emotive behavior therapy (REBT) maintains that it is important for clients to understand the role of beliefs in symptom development. The first step in doing this is to teach clients to distinguish between the As, Bs, and Cs of REBT, or the ABC model. "A" stands for activating events or eliciting stimuli. "B" stands for the beliefs, thoughts, and cognitions that people have in response to "A." "C" stands for the consequences that clients experience, and these can be of two types: emotional and behavioral. The consequences can be negative, disturbing emotional experiences, such as depression, anxiety, or dysfunctional anger as well as dysfunctional behavioral reactions such as avoidance, procrastination, or aggression. Remember, these consequences are the symptoms for which clients seek therapy.

It is important to teach clients to become aware of what the triggering, preceding events are and to clarify their emotional and behavioral consequences related to these events. The clients' symptoms, which often are what lead them to seek out therapy, will be the emotional and behavioral consequences that are triggered by their beliefs about the activating events that precede them. The final component of the REBT ABC

https://doi.org/10.1037/0000334-003

Deliberate Practice in Rational Emotive Behavior Therapy, by M. D. Terjesen, K. A. Doyle, R. A. DiGiuseppe, A. Vaz, and T. Rousmaniere

model is that of beliefs. People usually have several thoughts and beliefs about an activating event, and these occur almost simultaneously with or after the activating events, and before or simultaneously with the consequences. These beliefs include attributions, inferences, conclusions, perceptions, expectations, demands, and evaluations about the activating events or about the people who committed the activating events, which could be the clients themselves or others.

By becoming aware of the relationship between the activating events, the beliefs the client has about them, and the client's dysfunctional emotional and behavioral consequences, the therapist sets the stage for the REBT skills taught in therapy. This skill focuses on effectively developing the clinician's ability to communicate the ABC model of REBT to clients. By providing clear education about the ABC model, we hope the clinician sets the foundation for the skills that involve the beliefs and consequences.

SKILL CRITERIA FOR EXERCISE 1

1. Using content from the client's statement, educate the client on the REBT ABC model.
2. Check for the client's understanding of the REBT ABC model.

Examples of Therapists Using Psychoeducation About Rational Emotive Behavior Therapy's ABC Model

Example 1

CLIENT: [*angry*] My boss really makes me angry when she doesn't respond to my repeated requests for guidance. I really can't stand this, and I want to tell her off. She always does this. So help me understand, how is this therapy going to work if she keeps doing this?

THERAPIST: Thanks for your question and your specific example. The REBT model of therapy focuses on the relationship between situations, beliefs, and feelings and behaviors. You describe the situation of your boss not responding, which in REBT we call the activating event, or A, and at point C, you report feelings of anger and the thought of telling her off, which is the behavior. In REBT, these feelings and behaviors are the consequences, or Cs. In REBT, we focus on the beliefs or thoughts about that situation that lead to those feelings and behaviors and try to see if those beliefs are illogical or unhelpful. This middle step is called the beliefs or B in the ABC model. If we work on getting you to think differently, maybe you will feel something different from and healthier than the anger you describe even if she does continue to do this. (Criterion 1) Does that make sense to you? (Criterion 2)

Example 2

CLIENT: [*anxious*] I am so scared watching the news. The new COVID variant is spreading all over. Hearing the news makes me anxious and stops me from doing anything. I am vaccinated, and I am not worried about getting sick. But I feel sure that the economy will collapse again, and that makes me anxious that we'll all be on lockdown. We couldn't go out again. I couldn't go to work and couldn't see people. I couldn't stand that happening again. I have been trying to work from home, and when I get anxious, I stop working. I just stare at the TV. I know I cannot control what is going to happen, but what do I do about this anxiety?

THERAPIST: I hear that you are experiencing anxiety and the primary event that you get upset about is the spread of the COVID variant. You are correct that you cannot control what may happen, but maybe we can work on the anxiety. In REBT, we look at the situation, or the activating event, or A, which in this case is the spread of the variant. The emotional consequence, or C, is the feeling of anxiety and your behaviors—you watch more news, you freeze, and do nothing. The beliefs, or B, are the beliefs that you have about this potential COVID spread. In REBT, we work on looking at whether these beliefs are helpful, logical, and true, and, if not, then work on changing them to more rational or healthier beliefs. (Criterion 1) Does this approach make sense? (Criterion 2)

Example 3

CLIENT: [*depressed*] I want to talk about my recent experience with my partner. I come home after a hard day and try to talk to her. And what do I get? Nothing. She completely ignores me. She doesn't even say hello or lift her eyes from her iPad. I feel so depressed. Like I do not even matter to her. I am a nobody! She totally ignored me. Even when I spoke to her, she **ignored** me. I felt like I was a total loser. Not only was I depressed, I was a little angry too. I was shocked, then I was mad and raised my voice and sulked and banged things. I said, "Hey who do you think you are? I don't deserve this treatment." What am I supposed to do in these situations? How can this therapy help me?

THERAPIST: That sounds very disappointing, and your question is an important one. Let's try to break the situation down into its parts and put it into the ABC model of REBT. The event that triggered your depression, sadness, and some anger was her not speaking to you and focusing on her iPad. In REBT, we call this triggering event the A for activating event. You reported that when this happened, you experienced three emotions—depression, sadness, and some anger—and that you yelled at her and sulked around the house. These emotional and behavioral responses we call the C or the consequences. Now, people often have beliefs and thoughts about the events that upset them. In REBT, that is our focus, looking at these Bs for beliefs, we work together to see if they are accurate and helpful and if they make sense. (Criterion 1) Does that make sense to you? That we will work on changing these emotions and behaviors by focusing on your beliefs about her behavior? (Criterion 2)

INSTRUCTIONS FOR EXERCISE 1
Step 1: Role-Play and Feedback
• The client says the first beginner client statement. The therapist **improvises** a response based on the skill criteria.   • The trainer (or if not available, the client) provides **brief** feedback based on the skill criteria.   • The client then repeats the same statement, and the therapist again improvises a response. The trainer (or client) again provides brief feedback.
Step 2: Repeat
• Repeat Step 1 for all the statements **in the current difficulty level** (beginner, intermediate, or advanced).
Step 3: Assess and Adjust Difficulty
• The therapist completes the Deliberate Practice Reaction Form (see Appendix A) and decides whether to make the exercise easier or harder or to repeat the same difficulty level.
Step 4: Repeat for Approximately 15 Minutes
• Repeat Steps 1 to 3 for at least 15 minutes.   • The trainees then switch therapist and client roles and start over.

Now it's your turn! Follow Steps 1 and 2 from the instructions.

Remember: The goal of the role-play is for trainees to practice improvising responses to the client statements in a manner that (a) uses the skill criteria and (b) feels authentic for the trainee. **Example therapist responses for each client statement are provided at the end of this exercise. Trainees should attempt to improvise their own responses before reading the example responses.**

BEGINNER-LEVEL CLIENT STATEMENTS FOR EXERCISE 1
Beginner Client Statement 1
[Angry] So my coworker comes by with a new project for us to do, and he has convinced the boss that we all should do this. Now, I will never get to my work. I am so furious at him. He should just be like one of us and stop trying to impress the boss with plans that involve everyone else. I was so angry that I cursed at my coworker in front of others. How am I supposed to deal with this?
Beginner Client Statement 2
[Depressed] I feel so depressed and down. I just got my screenplay rejected. I just have these thoughts running through my mind. I will never be able to write good work. I will never be good enough to have my work performed; I will never be successful at anything, which will make me a total failure. So, I'm just avoiding doing any writing these days—or anything else. Help me understand what we will work on to make me feel less depressed and push forward.
Beginner Client Statement 3
[Guilty] Last week, I had to work, and I couldn't be there to take my mom to the hospital for her chemotherapy appointment. She was scared and did not feel so good about my cousin bringing her instead of me. I should have been there for her and gotten out of work. Not being there for her really makes me a loser. I deserve to pay for not helping her. I felt so guilty that I couldn't get up the courage to go see her for 2 days. So help me understand, how is this therapy going to work as I already screwed up?
Beginner Client Statement 4
[Anxious] There is this big project at work. Whoever does the best work will get the promotion. I'm not sure that I'll do so well because my team is full of talented people. I am anxious that I won't make a good impression. It will be awful if I don't get the promotion and show what a loser I am. When I feel anxious, I just put off doing any work. How does REBT work?
Beginner Client Statement 5
[Jealous] My partner does not seem to be talking to me much anymore. And when she does, she's always talking about this guy at her work. I think she is more interested in him than me. I feel so jealous. If I lost her, I couldn't stand it. I feel hurt, and just don't talk to her or I withdraw. I'm uncertain that talking about this will change things.

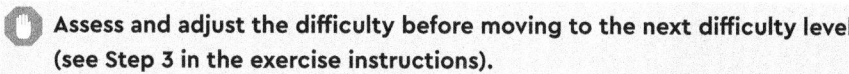 **Assess and adjust the difficulty before moving to the next difficulty level (see Step 3 in the exercise instructions).**

INTERMEDIATE-LEVEL CLIENT STATEMENTS FOR EXERCISE 1

Intermediate Client Statement 1

[Angry] I had an excellent plan for how I would get all my work done. But the bosses sent a work team who were such losers. They didn't follow any of my instructions, and I had to stay on them or they would take too many breaks. They were such losers. I really lost my temper; I was so angry. Does your therapy let me just be OK with them being so incompetent? Not sure I want that approach.

Intermediate Client Statement 2

[Depressed] I really tried to understand this new writing project I was assigned. But I felt it was so hard. I just couldn't make any progress on it. I thought I was such a loser for not getting it. I just stayed in bed for 2 days and got nothing done. How does your therapy help?

Intermediate Client Statement 3

[Guilty] I feel so guilty about going on vacation. I go on vacations so infrequently. I should have been more careful with my money. I am such a fool for making that mistake. Now I'm just spending money again like it doesn't matter. I already messed up. I have talked about this before, but no change happens, either with the money or the guilt. What will be different this time?

Intermediate Client Statement 4

[Anxious] I have some new assignments at work. Some things that I have never done before, and I get worried that I will screw this up and it will be awful. I am so anxious, and I just freeze when I start to work. I know you cannot make these assignments easier for me, but how will your approach to therapy help me?

Intermediate Client Statement 5

[Jealous] I thought I was pretty secure at my job. But there is a new person in the department who has been doing great work, and everyone notices the skills she displays. I feel I could lose my manager position to her. That would be awful. Can we discuss how best to manage my jealousy so I do as good of a job as I can?

 Assess and adjust the difficulty before moving to the next difficulty level (see Step 3 in the exercise instructions).

ADVANCED-LEVEL CLIENT STATEMENTS FOR EXERCISE 1

Advanced Client Statement 1

[Angry] I am trying to rest and watch TV, and my wife started nagging me about watching TV and not doing something useful. She won't stop talking about why I should do something else. She will nag me all day, and yesterday I yelled at her. I feel that she should understand that my responsibilities are done since I retired. She doesn't understand me. How can your approach to therapy help me change her?

Advanced Client Statement 2

[Depressed] I have so much work to do, and I just can't keep a schedule that allows me to do all the work and be with my partner. I feel there is not enough time to do everything and have time for myself. I really believe I should be able to figure this out. Others seem to be able to do so. I feel so depressed that I took a mental health day. Now, I am even further behind. This is hopeless and I can't do anything about it. I don't even know if I have time for therapy.

Advanced Client Statement 3

[Guilty] I have been thinking about the effect my drinking has had on my family. I feel I have been a terrible parent and spouse. I feel I am such a loser, and I am so guilty. When I get these feelings, I just drink some more and get nothing done. What will your approach to therapy do to help me deal with this problem?

Advanced Client Statement 4

[Anxious] I have to do this big presentation at work. I know it will not come across well. I feel the people will just not like my presentation, and I will make some mistakes. It will be awful. I get shaky each time I think of it. That results in me delaying and not getting my presentation done. I assume you won't give me feedback on my presentation, but how can therapy help?

Advanced Client Statement 5

[Jealous] It was such an awful experience to see my partner flirting with another guy. I have always been insecure and felt that no one could really love me. I feel so messed up inside. I imagine my partner will find someone better than me. When I feel this way, I just say hurtful things to my partner to see if he really loves me. Can your therapy approach help me not give in to my jealous urges?

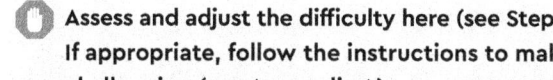 **Assess and adjust the difficulty here (see Step 3 in the exercise instructions). If appropriate, follow the instructions to make the exercise even more challenging (see Appendix A).**

Example Therapist Responses: Psychoeducation About Rational Emotive Behavior Therapy's ABC Model

Remember: Trainees should attempt to improvise their own responses before reading the example responses. **Do not read the following responses verbatim unless you are having trouble coming up with your own responses!**

<table>
<tr><td align="center">**EXAMPLE RESPONSES TO BEGINNER-LEVEL
CLIENT STATEMENTS FOR EXERCISE 1**</td></tr>
<tr><td>*Example Response to Beginner Client Statement 1*</td></tr>
<tr><td>That does sound like it can be difficult. In REBT, we look at each emotional episode in an ABC model. Let me explain this using your example, and we can see whether this is an approach you think will be helpful. It sounds like the activating event, or A, was when your coworker got the boss to assign a new project and your emotional consequence, or C, was becoming furious and the behavioral consequences were you cursing at him. In REBT, we try to change the C—in this case, anger—by focusing on the B, the beliefs you are having, which were that he should become one of the team members and stop trying to impress the boss. (Criterion 1) Do you understand that by working on changing your belief, we can assist you in controlling your anger? (Criterion 2)</td></tr>
<tr><td>*Example Response to Beginner Client Statement 2*</td></tr>
<tr><td>I think it's great that you don't want to feel depressed and want to push forward. Sadness may be a better emotion for you to experience in this context. We will work on getting you to recognize how your beliefs about these rejections lead you to feel depressed and avoid writing. In REBT, we follow an ABC model. First, we identify the situation, trigger, or what we call the A for activating event, which was getting the rejection of your screenplay. Your emotional reaction was feeling depressed and your behavioral reaction of avoidance. We call these consequences or Cs. Now, if we cannot change the situation and want to work on changing the consequences that we experience, we will look at changing some of your unhealthy Bs or beliefs that come between the As and Cs. In this episode, it is your thinking that you will never be a good writer, never have your work performed, and never be successful at anything and that would make you a total failure. (Criterion 1) Do you understand that if we focus on your beliefs, we will put you in a better position to feel sad instead of depressed and push forward to continue writing? (Criterion 2)</td></tr>
<tr><td>*Example Response to Beginner Client Statement 3*</td></tr>
<tr><td>I understand the guilt you are experiencing, and I'm hopeful that together we can help you think differently about this to then feel differently as well. This type of therapy looks at the relationship among situations, thoughts or beliefs, and consequences and we use what is called an ABC model. Here, the emotional consequence, or C, is the strong guilt that you felt. The event or the situation that started it, which we call the activating event or A, was your not being able to take your mom for her chemotherapy treatment. You reported several thoughts or irrational beliefs that are associated with the guilt: "I should have taken her no matter what, and I am a loser for not taking her." These beliefs are what we consider the Bs in the ABC model. (Criterion 1) Does how I conceptualized the problem help you understand that our approach will focus on changing those beliefs to more realistic, healthy, and logical ones? (Criterion 2)</td></tr>
</table>

Example Response to Beginner Client Statement 4

This therapy works by doing an ABC analysis of this situation to construct a plan of action. The A is the activating event, and here it is this special project that needs to be done. You describe that you are experiencing a significant amount of anxiety about this project, and that leads you to avoid working on it. The anxiety and avoidance would be the consequence, or C. This anxiety seems instigated by beliefs you have. You think that people's performance on this project will determine who gets the next promotion, and it would be "awful" if it was not you; this would further confirm that you are a loser. These are the beliefs or Bs. We work on helping you identify the unhealthy Bs and then changing them to help change your Cs. (Criterion 1) Does this conceptualization and our plan of action make sense? (Criterion 2)

Example Response to Beginner Client Statement 5

You sound very upset, and I understand your reluctance about talking and whether it would help. To explain the process of the therapy I do, let me try to fit this situation into an ABC analysis to organize a plan. The A, or the activating event, is the situation where your partner is talking to you much less than before. You then think she is interested in another guy, and if this is true you might lose her, and you could "not stand" that happening. These are called the beliefs or Bs. As a result of the event and, more importantly, your beliefs about the event, you feel jealous, and you then talk to her less as well. These are the consequences or Cs. If we want to work on changing how you feel and what you do, we would target those unhealthy beliefs for change. (Criterion 1) Does that approach to therapy make sense to you? (Criterion 2)

EXAMPLE RESPONSES TO INTERMEDIATE-LEVEL CLIENT STATEMENTS FOR EXERCISE 1

Example Response to Intermediate Client Statement 1

That is a good question, and it might be helpful for me to describe how REBT works to address your question. REBT tries to understand an emotional episode in an ABC model. In your situation, the A, or activating event, was that the workers on the project that you supervised did not follow directions. They took too many breaks, and you had to stay on them to get work done. The C, or consequence, of this situation was that you became angry and lost your temper. But there is a middle step between the A and the C, and that is the B in this model, which are your beliefs about the workers. The beliefs you expressed were that they were "losers," and I imagine you might have thoughts like you "cannot stand" this, and the bosses "should not" have sent you this team of losers. Although we cannot change what happened or how effective the workers are, we can work on changing your beliefs to ones that are healthier for you. That does not mean thinking their incompetence is OK, but rather, you can develop a more healthy, realistic way of thinking. (Criterion 1) Do you understand that we will focus on your beliefs that cause these emotional responses and what thoughts would help you? (Criterion 2)

Example Response to Intermediate Client Statement 2

Let me explain how this therapy works, and then we can discuss whether you think it would help you. To begin, the approach starts by taking each emotional episode and conceptualizing it into an ABC model. Your situation, the activating event, or A, is that you were assigned a new project that was very difficult. The belief, or B, you have about this project was that you were a "loser." These beliefs lead to your behavioral consequence, or C, that you stayed in bed for 2 days and did no work. There probably also is a feeling or emotion that you experienced when all this happened. In REBT, we work on looking at whether your beliefs are healthy, logical, and accurate. (Criterion 1) Does this approach make sense to you? (Criterion 2)

Example Response to Intermediate Client Statement 3

You ask a good question: What will talking about this do that is different from before? The answer is both simple and complex. Talking about it most likely will not change what happened. We follow an ABC model to guide our treatment. The activating event, or A, is the situation you describe, that is you spending money that you do not have. The middle step is the Bs, or the beliefs you have that lead you to feel guilty, which is an emotional consequence or C. So we don't just talk about the problem, but we work on changing those beliefs, and if you changed them, we imagine you would feel something negative but less disturbed and maybe behave differently. That is what the process of REBT is all about. Together we look at challenging the beliefs about situations and try to see if we can develop a more realistic, sensible, helpful way of thinking. (Criterion 1) Does this approach sound different from what you did previously? More importantly, do you think this would help you? (Criterion 2)

Example Response to Intermediate Client Statement 4

You are right that I cannot make those assignments easier for you, but in REBT we would identify and examine the beliefs you have about the assignment that contribute to your anxiety and your tendency to freeze up. If we organize the elements of this story, the activating event, or A, is receiving new assignments at work; you report the C, or consequences, of the new assignments as feeling anxious and freezing up, stopping your work. These are the emotional and behavioral consequences. Our model proposes that the cause of the C is the middle step between the A and the C. That is the beliefs or Bs that you have about the event. We then look to see if these beliefs help you in any way and if they are accurate and make sense. If not, we try to change them. (Criterion 1) Do you understand how this approach would work and think it could help you? (Criterion 2)

Example Response to Intermediate Client Statement 5

It's great that you want to work on your jealousy. The REBT approach might be an effective avenue for treatment. REBT uses an ABC model. For each emotional episode, it identifies the consequence or C that you feel in situations. Here it is the jealousy you experience in situations. The activating event or A in the model is the situation where this new person at work is competent and other people notice; you worry that might result in their thinking of you as less competent. In addition to understanding the situation and the feelings, we look at the different beliefs, or Bs, you have about this situation. We examine whether these beliefs are accurate, make sense, or are helpful; if they are not, we then discuss how to change the beliefs and subsequently our feelings and behaviors. (Criterion 1) Do you understand the role that these beliefs play and how we would initially target them for change within this model? (Criterion 2)

EXAMPLE RESPONSES TO ADVANCED-LEVEL CLIENT STATEMENTS FOR EXERCISE 1

Example Response to Advanced Client Statement 1

Before we discuss any strategies for changing her and whether that is realistic, let me present another approach to therapy called REBT. In REBT, we analyze emotional episodes in an ABC model. The activating event, or A, is the event you are upset about. Here it is that you are watching TV and your wife tells you to do other things. She criticizes you for just lounging. You then experience several beliefs, the Bs that go between As and Cs. Here you think she won't stop, and she "should" understand that you don't have responsibilities since you retired. The consequence, or C, is that you yelled at her yesterday and what sounds like some anger. In this approach, we work to understand the interaction among the beliefs, the feelings, and the behaviors and together and move towards more healthy, realistic, and logical ways of thinking to assist you in experiencing healthier emotions and behaviors. (Criterion 1) While I understand that you really want her to change, do you understand that we will focus on your beliefs about her behavior to help you feel and act differently? (Criterion 2)

Example Response to Advanced Client Statement 2

I appreciate the challenges you are reporting, and maybe if I discuss the type of therapy I do, you can help make an informed decision if you think this will be worth your time. In REBT, we follow an ABC model. We work on understanding the relationship between what happens, the A or activating event; what you believe or think about what happens, referred to as the beliefs or Bs; and how you feel and act as a result of those beliefs, what we consider the consequences or Cs in the model. Here, you sound upset about the pressures between work and home with too much work for you to schedule and then not having enough time with your partner. The beliefs that you have about that sound like they are that you "should" be able to figure out your schedule as others seem to do. The emotional consequence is that you feel depressed. In REBT, we work on changing those beliefs to more functional, logical, and accurate ones. (Criterion 1) Do you understand the process of this therapy and how we will target these thoughts and beliefs that lead you to feeling depressed? (Criterion 2)

Example Response to Advanced Client Statement 3

From what you describe, it sounds like you want to know how REBT works and then determine whether you think this would help you. In REBT, we try to conceptualize difficulties within an ABC model: The A is the activating event or what happened, the B is the beliefs about that event, and the C is the consequences that result from these beliefs. The consequences are both the emotions you feel and the behaviors you do. It sounds like some of the beliefs you have are that you have been a terrible spouse and father, and you are such a "loser." These beliefs lead to a behavioral consequence—you drink more. In REBT, if we want to change the consequences, here the guilt and drinking, we work on changing the beliefs that lead to them. (Criterion 1) Does this approach make sense to you? (Criterion 2)

Example Response to Advanced Client Statement 4

Great question: How can therapy help you? Well, let me discuss the approach I use, which is called REBT. And then you can tell me if you think it will help. Let's start by putting this emotional episode in the ABC format, which is how we conceptualize situations in REBT. The activating event, or A, is an event about which you are upset. In this case, it is that you have to make a presentation at work. Now you said you feel that others won't like your presentation, you will make some mistakes, and that this would be awful. These sentences sound like thoughts and beliefs to me, and that is the middle part of the ABC model—the beliefs. They are predictions and evaluations about what could happen. You then said that you delay getting your presentation done and that you feel shaky, which may be anxiety. These are the consequences, or Cs, that you are experiencing as a result of these beliefs. In REBT, we work together to determine if these beliefs make sense, are helpful, and are accurate. (Criterion 1) Was I clear in describing this model, and do you think this would be helpful for you? (Criterion 2)

Example Response to Advanced Client Statement 5

I think your motivation to give up your jealous urges is a good one. Let me discuss the model of therapy I use, and then we can see whether you think it will help you to work toward that goal. In REBT, we try to organize the elements of a situation like yours into an ABC model. The A, or activating event, is that you see your partner flirting with another guy. You then have certain ideas, such as imagining that your partner will find someone else and that this would be "awful" for you. That is the belief, or B. And when you think these things, you feel jealous and say hurtful things to him. These are the consequences, or Cs. If we want to change the consequences and not give in to your jealous urges, we work on changing your beliefs or thoughts. (Criterion 1) Did I describe this approach in a manner that is understandable, and do you think it will be helpful to managing your jealous urges? (Criterion 2)

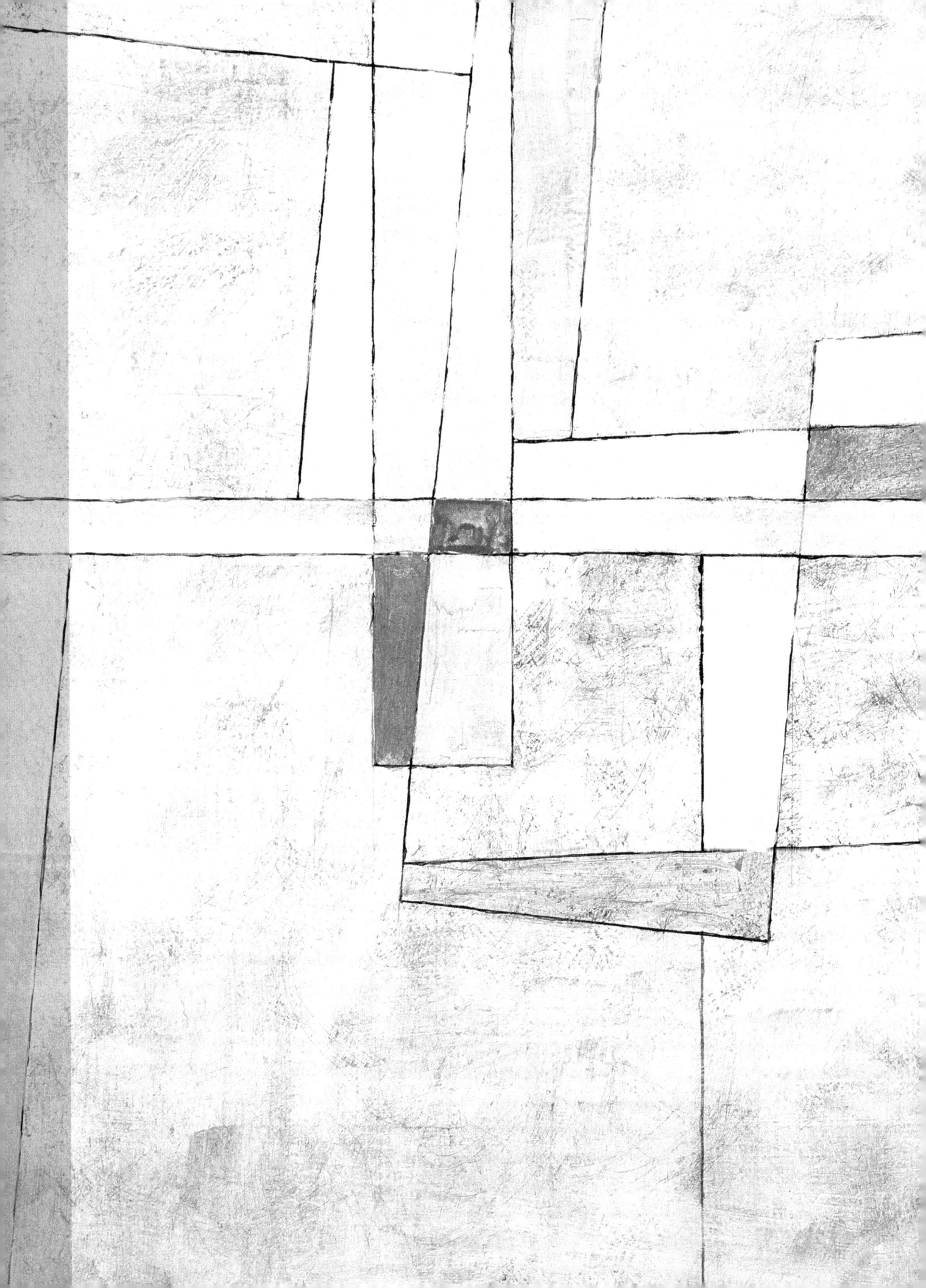

Psychoeducation About Dysfunctional Versus Functional Negative Emotions and Behaviors

Preparations for Exercise 2

1. Read the instructions in Chapter 2.

2. Download the Deliberate Practice Reaction Form and the Deliberate Practice Diary Form at https://www.apa.org/pubs/books/deliberate-practice-rational-emotive-behavior-therapy (see the "Clinician and Practitioner Resources" tab; also available in Appendixes A and B, respectively).

Skill Description

Skill Difficulty Level: Beginner

Our emotions serve as internal signals to us that a problem exists in our environment that requires our attention and action. Thus, we will always have some negative emotions because problems in life will always occur. Most psychotherapies address the emotional goals of therapy as the reduction in the intensity of the client's emotions. This is usually conceptualized as a reduction on the emotions Subjective Units of Discomfort (SUDs) scale—that is, how upsetting and strong was the negative emotional experience for an individual client. Psychotherapy is expected to produce less intense SUDs, such as less intense feelings of depression, anger, guilt, and other targeted emotions. Suggesting that the client work to achieve a reduction in the intensity of the emotion could be experienced as invalidating and is not consistent with the rational emotive behavior therapy (REBT) model. Significant negative events happen to everyone and usually elicit strong emotional reactions. Therefore, REBT teaches that negative emotions are part of life and that we will always have them. Given the certainty of negative life events, the question is then which negative emotions we will experience and can we aim toward experiencing healthier more adaptive negative emotions. A reduction in the intensity

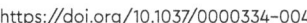

https://doi.org/10.1037/0000334-004

Deliberate Practice in Rational Emotive Behavior Therapy, by M. D. Terjesen, K. A. Doyle, R. A. DiGiuseppe, A. Vaz, and T. Rousmaniere

of the emotion can imply to the client that such events are not so important. REBT makes a crucial distinction between the qualitative types of emotions that people can experience. For each family of emotions, REBT postulates there are at least two (and probably more) emotional experiences that a person can have. Some of these emotions are negative, unhealthy, disturbed reactions to an adverse activating event. Others are healthy, adaptive emotional reactions to an adverse activating event.

Unhealthy, disturbed, negative emotions (UNEs) can vary in intensity from moderately strong to very intense. They interfere with the person achieving their goals. They lead to the person narrowing their focus on the catastrophic nature of the problem rather than engaging in problem solving of solutions or applying coping strategies. They elicit behavioral inflexibility. That is, the responses that people have to these activating events are often limited to the things they have done in the past that often do not work. Healthy, nondisturbed, negative emotions (HNEs) can have moderate intensity. They allow one to focus on generating solutions to the problem, and they elicit behavioral flexibility so that the person can focus on behaviors that resolve their problem.

The REBT theory proposes that irrational beliefs lead to UNE and dysfunctional behaviors, whereas rational beliefs lead to HNE and adaptive behaviors. Given this theory, a negative activating event and rational thinking will result in a healthy, adaptive, negative emotion. Thus, the emotional goal of REBT is not a weaker or less intense emotion, nor a neutral emotion, but a negative emotion that motivates action and helps us focus on problem solving and coping.

A. Ellis (1994) listed the disturbed emotions with their corresponding healthy, adaptive, negative emotions. Thus, REBT works with clients to change depression to sadness or disappointment, to change anxiety to apprehension or concern, and to change guilt to remorse or regret. The emotions of anger and jealousy that we use in the exercises in this book present some special problems. The word "anger" in English can be used to convey adaptive and maladaptive variations of that emotion. Ellis often said that we would clinically change anger to annoyance. However, suggesting to a client that they feel annoyed at a major transgression, such as when they experience anger with their assailant or an insulting, racist person, can come across as invalidating. Perhaps a qualitatively different type of anger would be a better goal, and we can teach a client to go from destructive or clinical anger to adaptive motivating anger. Jealousy and an adaptive alternative emotional response present another problem because the English language does not have a word for adaptive jealousy. However, if one thought their romantic partner could leave them for another, they could feel concern that would motivate them to treat the partner better to keep them or prepare to live apart from them with as little distress as possible.

These problems of language are inherent in the conceptualization of unhealthy and healthy emotions. This problem will present differently for those who are conducting psychotherapy in languages other than English. We recommend that before you attempt to do REBT in a language other than English, you stop and contemplate the emotional vocabulary of your language and identify what words distinguish unhealthy versus healthy emotions in each of the basic families of negative emotions such as sadness, anger, fear, guilt, disgust, and shame.

Special Considerations for Performing This Exercise

The skill criteria represent three microskills that clinicians need to learn to educate clients properly about UNEs versus HNEs and their associated behaviors. Further, much like in many of the other exercises you will do, we provide different levels of client prompts to challenge the reader. At the beginner level, the clients provide information about how their UNE is dysfunctional. At the intermediate level, the clients state that they want to keep their UNE. At the advanced level, the client expresses some doubts about the advantages of the alternative emotion. The skill criteria remain the same across difficulty levels, but the client prompts vary in complexity to challenge the reader to consider how best to address these concerns and meet the skill criteria.

SKILL CRITERIA FOR EXERCISE 2

1. Teach the client that their UNE interferes with achieving their goals and elicits behaviors that are dysfunctional.
2. Teach the client an alternative HNE that helps them achieve their goals and elicits adaptive behaviors.
3. Propose that the goal of therapy be to replace a UNE with an HNE.

Examples of Therapists Using Psychoeducation About Dysfunctional Versus Functional Negative Emotions and Behaviors

Example 1

CLIENT: [*angry*] After all the favors I did for my brother, you would think he would show some appreciation and help me when I needed a hand. I am always helping him, and when I needed help moving, he is too busy because he has to go dancing. I am so furious. I really told him off and cursed him out good! I still have not spoken to him. And when the move was over, I invited the family over to see my new place. I invited everyone but him.

THERAPIST: It sounds like the unhealthy emotion you were experiencing was extreme fury and anger with your brother when he did not help you move. When you were angry, you cursed him out and excluded him from a family social event. (Criterion 1) The REBT solution is not to feel neutral toward your brother, as he often disappoints you. Could you imagine feeling an adaptive anger or annoyance that recognizes his inconsiderate behavior but does not consume you? This more functional anger would allow you to be aware that he will disappoint you and help you plan to protect yourself without discarding the relationship altogether. (Criterion 2) Do you think it's possible that we could work at replacing your destructive anger with this healthy negative emotion like constructive anger? (Criterion 3)

Example 2

CLIENT: [*anxious*] I am so scared watching the news. The new COVID-19 variant is spreading all over. Hearing the news makes me anxious and stops me from doing anything. I am vaccinated and I am not worried about getting sick. But I think that the economy will collapse again, and it makes me anxious that we will be on lockdown. I have been trying to work from home, but when I get anxious, I stop working. I just stare at the TV. I don't do work and I don't do any chores. I am a basket case.

THERAPIST: So, the dysfunctional unhealthy negative emotion you are experiencing is anxiety that immobilizes you, and the anxiety leads to behaviors that do not help you.

(Criterion 1) Another lockdown would be bad, and it makes sense to have some negative emotions about it. In REBT, we work to replace the anxiety with some type of apprehension that recognizes a problem but allows you to focus on what you can do about it. (Criterion 2) Would you agree that we can focus our session on changing your unhealthy anxiety to a healthier adaptive negative emotion, such as apprehension or concern? (Criterion 3)

Example 3

CLIENT: [*depressed*] I want to talk about my recent experience with my partner. I come home after work and go to talk to her. What do I get back from her? Nothing! She completely ignores me. She doesn't say hello or lift her eyes up from her iPad. I felt so depressed. The more depressed I got, the more I just thought about how awful it is to be ignored by her. My depression just overcame me, and I cried. When I get depressed, I just go to my room and binge watch some shows and avoid doing things that would be good for me, like thinking about fixing the problem to help me.

THERAPIST: Your unhealthy negative emotional reaction to her ignoring you was depression. The depression does not help you cope with the situation. In fact, you just continued to ruminate about the events. (Criterion 1) Also, your depression leads you to avoid speaking to her or trying to find out what is going on in the relationship. (Criterion 1) One of the goals of REBT is to work to replace the emotional experience of depression with sadness because sadness might lead you to do something to resolve the situation with her or cope better. (Criterion 2) Would you agree that we could work at replacing the unhealthy negative emotion of depression with the healthier negative emotion of sadness? (Criterion 3)

INSTRUCTIONS FOR EXERCISE 2

Step 1: Role-Play and Feedback

- The client says the first beginner client statement. The therapist **improvises** a response based on the skill criteria.
- The trainer (or if not available, the client) provides **brief** feedback based on the skill criteria.
- The client then repeats the same statement, and the therapist again improvises a response. The trainer (or client) again provides brief feedback.

Step 2: Repeat

- Repeat Step 1 for all the statements **in the current difficulty level** (beginner, intermediate, or advanced).

Step 3: Assess and Adjust Difficulty

- The therapist completes the Deliberate Practice Reaction Form (see Appendix A) and decides whether to make the exercise easier or harder or to repeat the same difficulty level.

Step 4: Repeat for Approximately 15 Minutes

- Repeat Steps 1 to 3 for at least 15 minutes.
- The trainees then switch therapist and client roles and start over.

Now it's your turn! Follow Steps 1 and 2 from the instructions.

Remember: The goal of the role-play is for trainees to practice improvising responses to the client statements in a manner that (a) uses the skill criteria and (b) feels authentic for the trainee. **Example therapist responses for each client statement are provided at the end of this exercise. Trainees should attempt to improvise their own responses before reading the example responses.**

BEGINNER-LEVEL CLIENT STATEMENTS FOR EXERCISE 2
Beginner Client Statement 1
[Angry] My coworker created a new project for us to do, and he has convinced the boss that we all should do this. I was so angry that I cursed at my coworker. And I have not cooperated on the new project yet.
Beginner Client Statement 2
[Depressed] I feel so depressed and down. I just got my screenplay rejected. I have these thoughts running through my mind. I will never write decent work. I will never be good enough to have my work performed. I will never be successful at anything. So, I'm just avoiding thinking about it or doing any writing these days—or anything else.
Beginner Client Statement 3
[Guilty] Last week, I had to work, and I couldn't be there to take my mom to the hospital for her chemotherapy. She was scared and didn't feel so good about my cousin bringing her instead of me. I should have been there for her and gotten out of work. I felt so guilty. When I feel guilty, I can't get up the courage to face her, so although she is not well, I did not see her for 2 days.
Beginner Client Statement 4
[Anxious] There is this big project at work. Whoever does the best work will get the promotion. I'm not sure that I will do well because my team is full of talented people. I feel so anxious. When I feel anxious, I can't focus on the work and ruminate about doing poorly. Then I just put off doing any work.
Beginner Client Statement 5
[Jealous] My partner does not talk to me much anymore. When she does, she talks about this guy at work. She is more interested in him than me. I feel so jealous. When I feel jealous, I just ruminate about her faults and don't talk to her. I sulk or withdraw, and I make sarcastic comments.

 Assess and adjust the difficulty before moving to the next difficulty level (see Step 3 in the exercise instructions).

INTERMEDIATE-LEVEL CLIENT STATEMENTS FOR EXERCISE 2
Intermediate Client Statement 1
[Angry] The team I had to work with that day were such losers. They didn't follow my instructions, and I had to stay on them. Yes, I know I lose my temper. I am here to work on my anger because it has gotten me in trouble at work, but anger is the only emotion that will help me manage those guys, and I can't imagine another way to feel.
Intermediate Client Statement 2
[Depressed] I feel depressed about this new writing project I was assigned. Yes, depression feels bad, and I have no energy to do anything. But I deserve to be depressed, and there is no other emotion to feel instead.
Intermediate Client Statement 3
[Guilty] I am feeling guilty about spending too much money on vacation. Even though I feel guilty, I keep spending too much money. However, I really think I should feel guilty for doing the wrong thing because guilt makes me take responsibility for making mistakes. I am not sure that less painful emotions would make me pay for my mistakes.
Intermediate Client Statement 4
[Anxious] I still feel anxious about the new assignments at work. When I am anxious, I just freeze rather than work. Part of me thinks anxiety is necessary to motivate me to work, and I can't think of another emotion to feel.
Intermediate Client Statement 5
[Jealous] I am still feeling jealous that this new person at work does such an excellent job and she will take my place as the manager. I watch everything she does and make sure I point out any errors she makes. I am developing a reputation as a critic. I am having a tough time not being jealous.

Assess and adjust the difficulty before moving to the next difficulty level (see Step 3 in the exercise instructions).

ADVANCED-LEVEL CLIENT STATEMENTS FOR EXERCISE 2
Advanced Client Statement 1
[Angry] I get angry when my wife nags me about watching TV and not doing something else. I feel that she should understand that my responsibilities are done since I retired. Don't I have a right to be angry if she keeps this up? So, I stay here and watch more TV just to make her angry and show her she can't control me.
Advanced Client Statement 2
[Depressed] I am so depressed that I will be laid off from work. It is the worst thing that could happen. I just want to do nothing but stay in bed. I know that depression is not helping me, but I can't imagine not being depressed. It would be impossible to feel just nothing about it.
Advanced Client Statement 3
[Guilty] I have been feeling so guilty about the effect my drinking has on my family. I have been a terrible parent and husband. But when I feel guilty, I am hopeless and just drink some more and get nothing done. But shouldn't I feel guilty about the harm I have caused?
Advanced Client Statement 4
[Anxious] I feel so anxious about this big presentation at work. When I am anxious, I just focus on my heart beating and the muscle tension and think of making a fool of myself. So, I delay working on my presentation. I can't imagine not being anxious.
Advanced Client Statement 5
[Jealous] I felt so jealous seeing my partner flirting with another guy. When I am jealous, I just think of him kissing the new person, which makes me feel worse. Or I say hurtful things to my partner to see if he really loves me. But that drives him away. How can I feel less jealous?

 Assess and adjust the difficulty here (see Step 3 in the exercise instructions). If appropriate, follow the instructions to make the exercise even more challenging (see Appendix A).

Example Therapist Responses: Psychoeducation Distinguishing Between Dysfunctional Negative Emotions and Maladaptive Behaviors and Healthy Negative Emotions and Functional Behaviors

Remember: Trainees should attempt to improvise their own responses before reading the example responses. **Do not read the following responses verbatim unless you are having trouble coming up with your own responses!**

**EXAMPLE RESPONSES TO BEGINNER-LEVEL
CLIENT STATEMENTS FOR EXERCISE 2**

Example Response to Beginner Client Statement 1

It sounds like your unhealthy emotional consequence was destructive anger. You felt furious and cursed out your colleague, and your failing to cooperate has not helped you at work. (Criterion 1) Imagine that you had some constructive healthy negative emotion, like constructive anger that allowed you to focus on how to fix the problem. (Criterion 2) In REBT, we work to try and help people to experience a healthier version of the negative emotion. Here, perhaps it would be a variant of anger that motivates you to state assertively your disagreement with his behavior or the new project. (Criterion 2) Would you agree to work in this session on replacing your destructive unhealthy negative emotion of anger with a healthy negative emotion, such as assertive, constructive anger? (Criterion 3)

Example Response to Beginner Client Statement 2

That is sad news. Based on what you described, your emotional experience, or consequence in REBT terms, is the unhealthy negative emotion of depression. This not only feels bad but it also stops you from thinking about writing or doing anything constructive or making any progress. (Criterion 1) The healthy negative emotion of sadness might be a better alternative emotional consequence. Sadness acknowledges the disappointment of the adverse event. However, it allows you to actively engage in problem solving and try to improve your manuscript. (Criterion 2) Do you agree that we could work on changing your unhealthy negative emotion of depression to the healthier negative emotion of sadness? (Criterion 3)

Example Response to Beginner Client Statement 3

When you did not take your mom to the hospital, your unhealthy emotional consequence was guilt, and this guilt did not help you resolve the issue with your mom. It interfered and led to your avoiding your mom for 2 days. (Criterion 1) In REBT, we work to replace the guilt with a healthier negative emotion such as remorse that would help you recognize your mistake and encourage you to fix it. Remorse would then help you do the right thing. (Criterion 2) How about we focus this therapy session on replacing the unhealthy guilt with an alternative healthy negative emotion, such as regret? (Criterion 3)

Example Response to Beginner Client Statement 4

Thinking about this project triggers the negative unhealthy emotional consequence of anxiety, and this emotion blocks your concentration and prevents you doing the work. (Criterion 1) The type of therapy we will do, REBT, works on helping you consider experiencing another negative emotion like apprehension or concern that we would call healthier because it acknowledges the high stakes and enhances your focus on the project, but does not overwhelm you. (Criterion 2) Further, a healthier negative emotion of apprehension or concern might motivate you to do the work. (Criterion 2) Should we work at replacing your anxiety with apprehension or concern? (Criterion 3)

Example Response to Beginner Client Statement 5

When your thoughts focus on ruminating about her talking to this other guy, your negative emotional consequence is jealousy. The jealousy leads to behavior that stresses the relationship. (Criterion 1) An alternative, healthier negative emotional experience of jealousy would feel more like concern. It would acknowledge that the relationship might be in trouble, but it could replace the rumination and fault finding with problem solving about how you could be closer to her and then lead to you behaving in a way that would support the relationship rather than what you are doing. (Criterion 2) Do you want to replace the unhealthy emotional consequence of jealousy with some healthy negative emotion, such as concern? (Criterion 3)

EXAMPLE RESPONSES TO INTERMEDIATE-LEVEL CLIENT STATEMENTS FOR EXERCISE 2

Example Response to Intermediate Client Statement 1

When you are working with the team and they don't follow instructions, your emotional consequence is the unhealthy negative emotion of anger. At other times, your anger has gotten you in trouble. (Criterion 1) Given this, it would be helpful to change that negative emotion of anger. In REBT, we would promote a healthy negative emotion instead of anger that may energize you to get results, focus on solutions, and speak in a firm, assertive, yet respectful manner to the workers. (Criterion 2) What would we call such a healthier, more adaptive negative emotion, and do we want to work toward that emotion? (Criterion 3)

Example Response to Intermediate Client Statement 2

When you face this writing project, your emotional consequence is the unhealthy negative emotion of depression, and that depression is your only choice of emotions. (Criterion 1) In REBT, we look to develop alternative healthier negative emotional reactions to depression, such as sadness. Sadness about the fact that the work is hard for you acknowledges the difficulty you experience. However, it leaves you with energy to focus on the task rather than thinking things are hopeless. (Criterion 2) You do not have to like things that you are sad about, but sadness allows you to go on with the rest of your life. (Criterion 2) Can you agree that we will spend our sessions changing your unhealthy negative depression to the healthier negative emotion of sadness? (Criterion 3)

Example Response to Intermediate Client Statement 3

You described that you spent too much money on vacation and that your emotional consequence is the negative unhealthy emotion of guilt. (Criterion 1) You are holding on to the guilt because you think it is necessary for you to suffer, yet the pain of the guilt has not helped you change your behavior. (Criterion 1) The theory of REBT proposes that we can replace the unhealthy negative emotion of guilt with a healthy negative emotion, such as regret. Regret is healthier because you still take responsibility for your behavior, and that emotion might allow you to focus on making corrections to your behavior. (Criterion 2) Do you want to keep the guilt or work toward feeling a healthier negative emotion of regret? (Criterion 3)

Example Response to Intermediate Client Statement 4

When you focus on the new work assignment you feel the emotional consequence of intense anxiety, which is unhealthy in that it blocks your concentrating on work. (Criterion 1) You think that anxiety is necessary because you cannot imagine a healthy, adaptive negative emotion to these events. The job is important to you, so you would not feel neutral about doing poorly. Instead of anxiety, the approach of REBT would work toward having you feel a healthy negative emotion, such as concern or apprehension. (Criterion 2) This feeling would acknowledge the importance of your work, yet it would not overwhelm you, so you would still be able to concentrate on the work. (Criterion 2) Does that make sense to you for something for us to work on? (Criterion 3)

Example Response to Intermediate Client Statement 5

Based on what you described, your emotional consequence to the recognition your new colleague gets is the unhealthy emotion of jealousy. Your jealousy gets you to pick at the colleague, and it backfires by giving you a reputation of a critic. This jealousy does not seem to be working for you. (Criterion 1) In the approach of REBT that I use, we work toward replacing the unhealthy negative emotion of jealousy with a healthy negative emotion, such as concern. Being concerned allows you to acknowledge the problem and focus on what you can do about it. It also stops you from being nasty or overly critical. (Criterion 2) Can we agree to work on replacing the unhealthy jealousy with healthy negative concern? (Criterion 3)

EXAMPLE RESPONSES TO ADVANCED-LEVEL CLIENT STATEMENTS FOR EXERCISE 2

Example Response to Advanced Client Statement 1

When your wife "nags" you, your emotional consequence is to feel the unhealthy negative emotion of anger. While you have the right to be angry and can justify it, it doesn't sound like it helps you resolve the conflict or lead to an adaptive behavior. (Criterion 1) Yes, your wife's behavior is unpleasant, and you can still have a negative but healthier emotion in reaction to her behavior. In REBT's work with anger, we would work on replacing your anger with some negative emotion like annoyance or an assertive anger that allows you to think through the problem before responding. (Criterion 2) Does it make sense to you to replace your critical anger with a negative but healthier emotion such as assertive anger? (Criterion 3)

Example Response to Advanced Client Statement 2

Your emotional consequence to being laid off is to feel depressed, and you are right that it would be impossible to feel neutral about such an important negative event. Depression has led to your lack of problem solving and your inactivity. (Criterion 1) The goal of REBT is not to go from depressed to neutral. But we could help you go from an unhealthy emotion like depressed to some healthier negative emotion, such as sadness. Sadness acknowledges that a major life crisis has occurred and helps you plan for it and allows you the energy to look for other work. (Criterion 2) Do you see how depression and sadness are different? (Criterion 3)

Example Response to Advanced Client Statement 3

When you think about the effect of your drinking your emotional consequence is the unhealthy negative emotion of guilt and it sounds like that guilt overwhelms you. It is good that you take responsibility and acknowledge the harm your drinking has done. However, guilt rarely leads people to change their bad behaviors. (Criterion 1) REBT works on replacing the guilt with a more adaptive, healthier negative emotion like regret. This emotion acknowledges your bad behavior and encourages you to stop the drinking and make amends to your family. (Criterion 2) Can you agree that we could work in our sessions on replacing your guilt with remorse? (Criterion 3)

Example Response to Advanced Client Statement 4

When you think about giving the presentation, your emotional consequence is anxiety. You think that this is the only emotion available to you. The anxiety gets you to focus on your unpleasant sensation rather than the presentation and it leads to inactivity. (Criterion 1) The type of work I do with REBT has clients work toward a different healthier negative emotion, say apprehension or concern. With apprehension or concern, you can feel a moderate level of arousal. You acknowledge the importance of the presentation and doing well. You are concerned about doing well but not frozen, and you can have heightened focus on what you need to do. And you can imagine sitting down and preparing. (Criterion 2) Can you agree that we could work at replacing the unhealthy negative emotion of anxiety with this healthier negative emotion of apprehension or concern that I described? (Criterion 3)

Example Response to Advanced Client Statement 5

When you see your partner talk to this guy, your emotional consequence is the negative unhealthy emotion of jealousy. Jealousy leads to dysfunctional behaviors, such as trying to get him to prove his love for you. It involves a host of beliefs about your partner being with another person that are upsetting and distracting. (Criterion 1) REBT recognizes that jealousy, regardless of how intense you feel it, is problematic. Perhaps the answer is to stop trying to feel less intense jealousy, but to replace jealousy with an alternative healthy negative emotion such as disappointment, which acknowledges the loss, stops the rumination, and develops plans to move on. (Criterion 2) Could you agree to working on replacing your jealousy with disappointment? (Criterion 3)

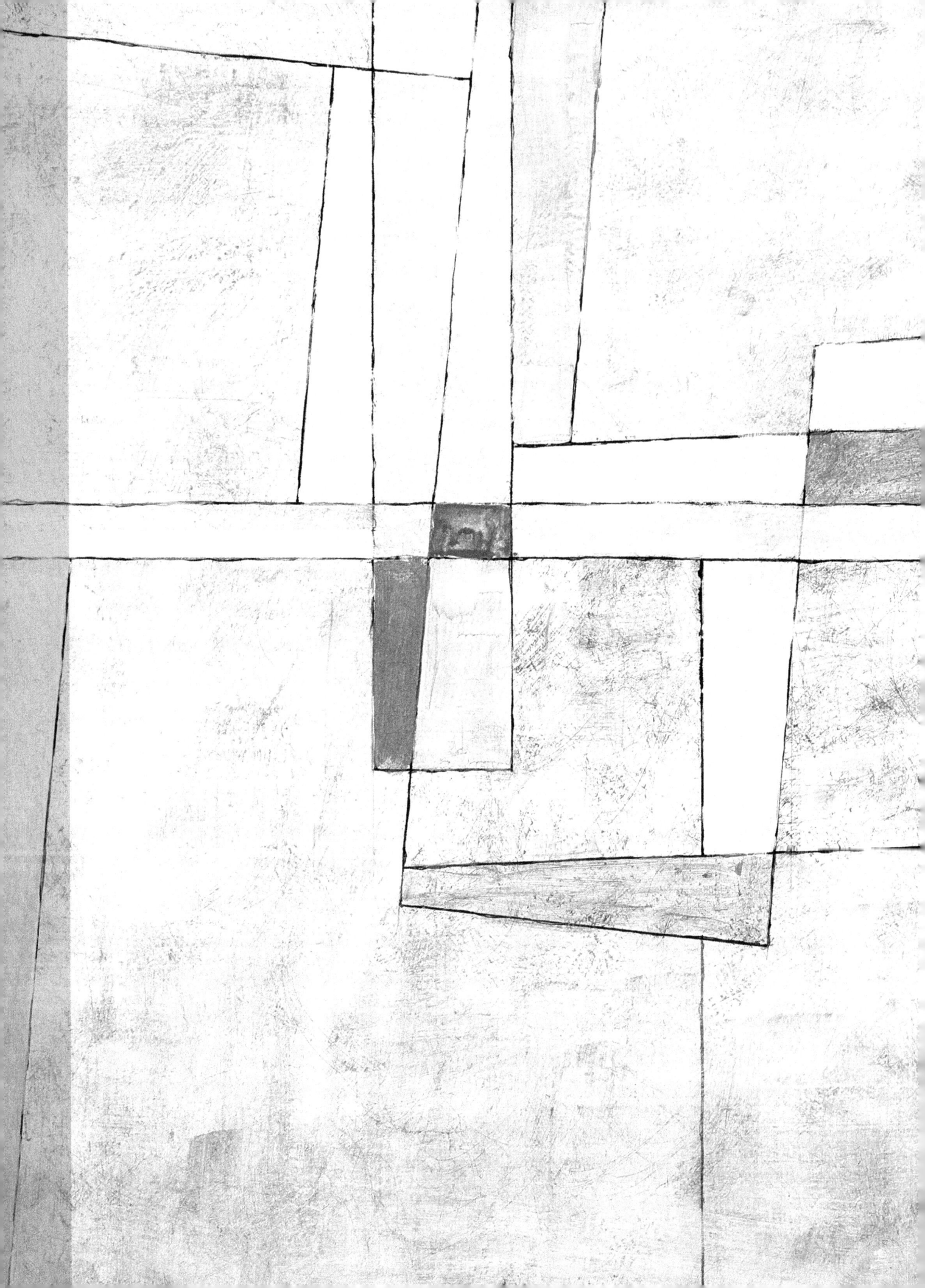

Agreement on the Session Goals

Preparations for Exercise 3

1. Read the instructions in Chapter 2.

2. Download the Deliberate Practice Reaction Form and the Deliberate Practice Diary Form at https://www.apa.org/pubs/books/deliberate-practice-rational-emotive-behavior-therapy (see the "Clinician and Practitioner Resources" tab; also available in Appendixes A and B, respectively).

Skill Description

Skill Difficulty Level: Beginner

For each session, the therapist wants to identify at least one goal that will be the focus of the session. Agreement on the goals of therapy is recognized as an important part of the therapeutic alliance that is a common factor for success in psychotherapy (Wampold & Imel, 2015). It is therefore an important part of rational emotive behavior therapy. We could not go on to the next steps of therapy (i.e., identifying and then disputing irrational beliefs) without specific goals. The therapist wants to clarify the client's emotional or behavioral goal that will be the focus of the session. Working with the client to understand the dysfunctional aspects of their emotions and behaviors to aversive stimuli helps prepare the client to work on targeting that goal for change and, more specifically, at the next step, the beliefs that lead to that negative consequence (the C of the ABC model covered in Exercise 1). We want to identify goals that are specific; therefore, we avoid vague or general goals, such as "I want to feel better." Clarifying the goal of the session involves asking questions that identify a specific unhealthy, disturbing emotion or a maladaptive behavior. Sometimes clients want to eliminate all emotional reactions, even healthy, adaptive emotions and/or behaviors that are

https://doi.org/10.1037/0000334-005

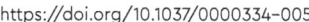

Deliberate Practice in Rational Emotive Behavior Therapy, by M. D. Terjesen, K. A. Doyle, R. A. DiGiuseppe, A. Vaz, and T. Rousmaniere

uncomfortable. These goals are unrealistic and might lead to dysfunctional outcomes if they were achieved.

In this exercise you will practice seeking agreement on the session goal of changing a specific emotional or behavioral consequence. The therapist should improvise a response to each patient statement following these skill criteria:

1. Clarify the content of the client's statement by translating it into a goal that represents the following:

   - Component A: The replacement of an unhealthy negative emotion (e.g., depression) with a healthy negative emotion (e.g., sadness). Agreement on an emotional goal represents not just the removal of a disturbed unhealthy negative emotion but replacing it with a negative albeit healthy adaptive emotional state. Thus, a goal might be stated in a compound sentence such as "I want to no longer experience social anxiety and replace it with experiencing apprehension or concern."

   - Component B: The reduction or elimination of a dysfunctional behavior (e.g., social avoidance) by the initiation or increase of a new adaptive behavior (e.g., social engagement). The behavioral goals targeted for change could be a behavioral excess that the client wants to decrease or eliminate or a behavioral deficit that the client wants to initiate or increase. Whenever possible, we encourage that you and the client state the behavioral goal in positive terms (e.g., "Help me approach more people to talk, even if I have some discomfort") as opposed to being negatively phrased (e.g., "Reduce my social anxiety"). Therefore, a behavioral goal might be "I want to increase the number of times I initiate talking with others even if I feel some apprehension, or concern about being rejected."

2. Ask for the client's agreement on a proposed goal: It is important that the therapist identifies the goals and that the client verbally agrees to them. Doing so facilitates collaboration and a positive therapeutic alliance, the quality of which has been shown to predict final treatment outcomes. Therefore, therapists finish their interventions by asking for the client's feedback or agreement on the proposed emotional or behavioral goal.

SKILL CRITERIA FOR EXERCISE 3

1. Clarify the client's statement by translating it into a goal that represents both of the following components:
   - Component A: The replacement of an unhealthy negative emotion (e.g., depression) with a healthy negative emotion (e.g., sadness)
   - Component B: The reduction or elimination of a dysfunctional behavior (e.g., social avoidance) by the initiation or increase of a new adaptive behavior (e.g., social engagement)
2. Ask for the client's agreement on a proposed goal.

Examples of Therapists Reaching an Agreement on the Session Goals

Example 1

CLIENT: [*angry*] I want to talk about my kids repeatedly not doing what I ask them to do. Recently, I got really angry, and I threw the remote control across the room. I don't want to have to parent this way, and I don't like what this is doing to my health. It took me maybe 2 hours to calm down that night.

THERAPIST: I know you want your kids to comply, but based on what you said that it does to you behaviorally and physically, would it make sense for us to focus on your experience of anger? And if you wanted to give up your anger, could you replace it with a healthier negative emotion such as frustration? (Criterion 1, Component A) Also, could we work on replacing the dysfunctional behavior of throwing things when angry with more adaptive behaviors? (Criterion 1, Component B) As you said, the anger preceded your behavior, do you agree that we will first work today on replacing your anger with frustration? (Criterion 2)

Example 2

CLIENT: [*anxious*] After that negative review from my boss, I put in my 2 weeks' notice at work. Right now, I am so anxious about finding a new job and paying for health insurance and paying off my student loans. When I try to sit down and start applying for jobs, a wave of anxiety comes over me, and I just avoid it and do anything else that is distracting.

THERAPIST: I hear considerable anxiety in what you are describing and some avoidance in applying for a job. So, to clarify, would you want to focus first on the unhealthy emotion of anxiety and replace it with a healthier negative emotion such as concern (Criterion 1, Component A) to help you then address the avoidance of applying for jobs? (Criterion 1, Component B) Because you have bills to pay, do you think it would be helpful today if we focus on replacing your anxiety so you can get started applying for jobs? (Criterion 2)

Example 3

CLIENT: [*depressed*] First, it was the hearing aids, then debilitating arthritis, and now they found a small tumor that they are going to remove. All of this is too much to handle. There are days that the depression is so significant I can't get out of bed, and I sometimes don't do the exercises that are recommended by my physical therapist for arthritis. People ask to get together, and I want to, but I just don't respond. Nothing works, and nothing will change my situation and how I feel.

THERAPIST: You mentioned feeling depressed and how that makes it hard to get out of bed, do the physical therapy exercises, and socialize. Would it be helpful for us to look at your experience of being depressed and move toward replacing it with sadness about your health? (Criterion 1, Component A) This might help us to address doing your physical therapy exercises and being more social. (Criterion 1, Component B) Are we in agreement that addressing your depression is the more important goal to begin with? (Criterion 2)

INSTRUCTIONS FOR EXERCISE 3

Step 1: Role-play and Feedback

- The client says the first beginner client statement. The therapist **improvises** a response based on the skill criteria.
- The trainer (or if not available, the client) provides **brief** feedback based on the skill criteria.
- The client then repeats the same statement, and the therapist again improvises a response. The trainer (or client) again provides brief feedback.

Step 2: Repeat

- Repeat Step 1 for all the statements **in the current difficulty level** (beginner, intermediate, or advanced).

Step 3: Assess and Adjust Difficulty

- The therapist completes the Deliberate Practice Reaction Form (see Appendix A) and decides whether to make the exercise easier or harder or to repeat the same difficulty level.

Step 4: Repeat for Approximately 15 Minutes

- Repeat Steps 1 to 3 for at least 15 minutes.
- The trainees then switch therapist and client roles and start over.

Now it's your turn! Follow Steps 1 and 2 from the instructions.

Remember: The goal of the role-play is for trainees to practice improvising responses to the client statements in a manner that (a) uses the skill criteria and (b) feels authentic for the trainee. **Example therapist responses for each client statement are provided at the end of this exercise. Trainees should attempt to improvise their own responses before reading the example responses.**

BEGINNER-LEVEL CLIENT STATEMENTS FOR EXERCISE 3
Beginner Client Statement 1
[Angry] My daughter stays on her phone all day and doesn't get her work done despite my reminding her. It usually ends up in a shouting match around 9:00 p.m., and then she stays up late and I have to stay up as well. She does this all the time, and it infuriates me. One night I threw her phone and cracked the screen.
Beginner Client Statement 2
[Depressed] Being alone sucks! Everyone is paired up and has a partner and no one wants to have a third wheel going places with them. With my kids off at school, my life has no purpose, I feel depressed, and I do nothing but sit at home and start pondering, "How did I end up here?" "What's wrong with me?" and "I am such a loser."
Beginner Client Statement 3
[Guilty] I put my mother in a retirement facility because she had medical needs that were beyond my capacity to deal with. I feel so incredibly guilty about this. I keep thinking I am a selfish person for doing this and maybe I should have tried harder with having her stay in my home. I can't even bring myself to visit her.
Beginner Client Statement 4
[Anxious] I have a few big decisions coming up about work and my relationship that result in my feeling crippling anxiety. I would like to know that I am making the right decision, but the lack of certainty leads me to feel anxious and my sleep is worse. My anxiety leads to inaction with these decisions and then they might be made for me instead of by me.
Beginner Client Statement 5
[Jealous] I organized this event and probably put more hours into it than anyone else. Yet I repeatedly watch the assistant events chair get all the credit for it. I am not sure if it is jealousy, envy, worry, or anger, but I think they might promote her to chair for this event next year. I have started secretly telling others how lazy she is.

 Assess and adjust the difficulty before moving to the next difficulty level (see Step 3 in the exercise instructions).

INTERMEDIATE-LEVEL CLIENT STATEMENTS FOR EXERCISE 3

Intermediate Client Statement 1

[Angry] My wife is so critical of me. Every night she has some complaint about something I did that she doesn't like. So, 2 nights ago, while I was working, she started criticizing me about my not helping with the dishes. I picked up my laptop and slammed it down on the table. It was ruined. And so was the stuff on the table. Perhaps I overreacted.

Intermediate Client Statement 2

[Depressed] I overcommitted myself at work and just don't think I can do all the things that I have on my plate. I really think I have messed up again, like I usually do. So, I just gave up and haven't done anything all week. I just surrendered.

Intermediate Client Statement 3

[Guilty] I know I have not been as good of a parent as I should have been to my youngest while she was growing up. I think I was really inattentive to her when she needed me . . . I was the worst, worthless person. Now I find myself doting. I will do anything for her. I bought the most ridiculous things to get her to forgive me. But I don't think it will work.

Intermediate Client Statement 4

[Anxious] I find myself thinking about how I am not going to get everything done and won't really do a good enough job. I keep going over my work to catch errors and make it better because I know others will think it is mediocre, which would be awful. I can't stop thinking about this and get so anxious and I can't stop checking my work. This worry affects my health and my relationship with the team.

Intermediate Client Statement 5

[Jealous] I am so upset that my partner will find someone else. She is great, attractive, smart, and talented. Almost any of the guys she works with are better than me. What does she see in a loser like me? I am always asking for reassurance. I need to keep our relationship.

 Assess and adjust the difficulty before moving to the next difficulty level (see Step 3 in the exercise instructions).

ADVANCED-LEVEL CLIENT STATEMENTS FOR EXERCISE 3

Advanced Client Statement 1

[Angry] My sister called me to ask me how work was going. I was midsentence discussing a really challenging colleague I work with, and she flipped the conversation to talk about herself. How could she do this again? I hung up on her, and my night was ruined.

Advanced Client Statement 2

[Depressed] Ever since the COVID pandemic started, I haven't been myself. I don't have the energy or desire to see friends, and I hate the way I look. Yesterday, I accidentally saw myself in the mirror and couldn't believe how much weight I've gained. I can't believe how I've let myself go. There is nothing I have to offer so I will never go out again.

Advanced Client Statement 3

[Guilty] I've been busy at work since I got that promotion. I come home late and just want to zone out and watch TV. Meanwhile, I haven't called my friend in several weeks who is going through a rough time right now. I keep asking myself, "Why aren't you just picking up the phone and calling her? What kind of a friend does this?"

Advanced Client Statement 4

[Anxious] I know we've been talking about me pushing myself to meet new people. Every week for homework it's the same thing, and I don't do it. I imagine going to a meetup group and not having anyone to talk to—or the reverse, I start talking to someone, and they look at me like I'm weird and quickly end the conversation.

Advanced Client Statement 5

[Jealous] Whenever my partner and I go out to this one restaurant we love, I notice he eyes the bartender throughout dinner. We were there last night, and he kept doing it, and I started grilling him, like asking if he was content with our relationship. I couldn't stop myself and I ruined the dinner. All I could think about for the rest of the evening was him looking at her.

 Assess and adjust the difficulty here (see Step 3 in the exercise instructions). If appropriate, follow the instructions to make the exercise even more challenging (see Appendix A).

Example Therapist Responses: Agreement on the Session Goals

Remember: Trainees should attempt to improvise their own responses before reading the example responses. **Do not read the following responses verbatim unless you are having trouble coming up with your own responses!**

EXAMPLE RESPONSES TO BEGINNER-LEVEL CLIENT STATEMENTS FOR EXERCISE 3
Example Response to Beginner Client Statement 1
It sounds like you are getting angry and doing behaviors like arguing and throwing phones that you don't want to do. To clarify our goals, would you want to work on feeling a more functional emotion, such as frustration, (Criterion 1, Component A) and work on being more assertive rather than aggressive with your words? (Criterion 1, Component B) Would you want to address your anger first, because it might organically help change those unhealthy behaviors? Could this be something you would agree to? (Criterion 2)
Example Response to Beginner Client Statement 2
To set a goal for this session, could we work on changing your depression to healthy sadness, (Criterion 1, Component A) which might then help you to become more active? (Criterion 1, Component B) Do we agree that it may be good to start with replacing your unhealthy depression first with a more functional emotion, such as sadness, and then move on to getting out more? (Criterion 2)
Example Response to Beginner Client Statement 3
You sound like you're feeling incredibly guilty for putting your mother in a retirement home, and now you are avoiding visiting her. If we had to set a goal to work on today, would it make sense to address the unhealthy guilt and replace it with a healthier emotion, such as regret? (Criterion 1, Component A) If you felt regret over what may have been a decision in your own self-interest, would you want to increase how frequently you visit her? (Criterion 1, Component B) Would today's goal be to work on changing your feelings of guilt and increase your visiting of her? (Criterion 2)
Example Response to Beginner Client Statement 4
This crippling anxiety you describe interferes with your sleep and leads to you not making potentially important decisions. Do you think changing that crippling anxiety to healthy concern would be helpful? (Criterion 1, Component A) Then you could start making some uncomfortable decisions. (Criterion 1, Component B) Do you agree that we should begin with your anxiety and hold off on actually making important decisions until you feel that healthy level of concern? (Criterion 2)
Example Response to Beginner Client Statement 5
You mention three emotions, but then you proposed that really it is this strong feeling of jealousy that leads you to sabotage her. Would working on changing those jealous feelings to disappointment be a goal you would want to focus on first? (Criterion 1, Component A) Then we could address your maladaptive behavior of sabotaging her? (Criterion 1, Component B) Since you sound like you want to keep this position, do we agree then that the goal is to replace that unhealthy jealousy with disappointment when the assistant events chair gets the credit? (Criterion 2)

EXAMPLE RESPONSES TO INTERMEDIATE-LEVEL CLIENT STATEMENTS FOR EXERCISE 3

Example Response to Intermediate Client Statement 1

You indicated that you believe your wife unfairly criticizes you, and you feel really angry and destroyed your property in an outburst. It sounds as if a good goal would be to work on changing those angry feelings and replacing them with some more functional emotions like disappointment or annoyance (Criterion 1, Component A) and then decrease the number of times you have outbursts and destroy property. (Criterion 1, Component B) Do you agree that our goal for today is to work on changing your anger to disappointment and reducing the aggressive outburst? (Criterion 2)

Example Response to Intermediate Client Statement 2

It sounds like you have overcommitted yourself and feel really depressed about it, which leads to a total shutdown of activity. Replacing that depression with regret (Criterion 1, Component A) would most likely help you problem solve about which tasks you can do. (Criterion 1, Component B) Would you agree that we will work on replacing depression with a more functional negative emotion and then begin working on some of your tasks? (Criterion 2)

Example Response to Intermediate Client Statement 3

It sounds like you are caught in a cycle where you feel guilty and then do things that are probably not good parenting. Examining that guilt and perhaps replacing it with a more adaptive negative emotion like regret (Criterion 1, Component A) and then parenting more effectively (Criterion 1, Component B) may be something that would be helpful for you. Do you agree that the goal of today's session is to replace your guilt with regret and then problem solve to be a more effective parent? (Criterion 2)

Example Response to Intermediate Client Statement 4

Your anxiety leads to all this checking behavior that stops you from finishing your work. I propose that for this session we work at replacing your anxiety with some concern about the quality of your work (Criterion 1, Component A) and reducing the checking behavior. (Criterion 1, Component B) What are your thoughts about us working on the anxiety and checking behavior in today's session? (Criterion 2)

Example Response to Intermediate Client Statement 5

Your jealousy leads to this clingy reassurance seeking. Perhaps we could work at replacing your dysfunctional jealousy with some type of concern (Criterion 1, Component A) and reduce the reassurance seeking. (Criterion 1, Component B) Do you think it would be a good idea for today's session for us to target the jealousy and reduce reassurance seeking? (Criterion 2)

EXAMPLE RESPONSES TO ADVANCED-LEVEL CLIENT STATEMENTS FOR EXERCISE 3

Example Response to Advanced Client Statement 1

When you say, "How could she do this again?" is it accurate to say that you then feel angry, get off the phone hastily, and your night is ruined? To clarify our goals, would you want to work on changing that dysfunctional anger toward your sister to a healthier emotion, such as annoyance, when she does this? (Criterion 1, Component A) And perhaps you might want to speak more politely to her when you say goodbye? (Criterion 1, Component B) Do you think it would be helpful to work on feeling annoyed but speaking more politely when she does this, rather than feeling angry? (Criterion 2)

Example Response to Advanced Client Statement 2

It sounds like when you say "There's nothing I have to offer" that you are saying you're inadequate or worthless and feel depressed as a result. Working toward a healthier but still negative emotion other than feeling depressed, such as sadness, can help you to make some changes that will improve your confidence (Criterion 1, Component A) while you also start engaging in healthier behaviors, like seeing your friends. (Criterion 1, Component B) So, could we work on moving from depression to sadness as a starting point because sadness doesn't paralyze you the way depression does? (Criterion 2)

Example Response to Advanced Client Statement 3

It sounds like you feel guilty about not calling your friend who is going through a rough time and that guilt is contributing to your continuing not to pick up the phone. In planning what we will work on, it sounds like you want to change that dysfunctional guilt to a more functional emotion, such as regret, (Criterion 1, Component A) and then replace the avoidance for not calling and take more action to contact your friend. (Criterion 1, Component B) Are we in agreement that we will address your guilt about not calling your friend first and replace it with healthy regret, and that might help motivate you to call her? (Criterion 2)

Example Response to Advanced Client Statement 4

It sounds like you're feeling anxious about being rejected, which leads you to avoid doing the homework we agree on. In setting goals, perhaps feeling a healthier negative emotion about the possibility of being rejected, such as concern, rather than that unhealthy anxiety (Criterion 1, Component A) would be helpful and might also make you more likely to complete the homework. (Criterion 1, Component B) To clarify, we are going to start by working on changing the anxiety to concern because you can see that it is the anxiety that, week after week, stops you from doing the homework. Does that seem like good place to start? (Criterion 2)

Example Response to Advanced Client Statement 5

What you describe sounds like you feel jealous when you see your boyfriend looking at this other woman. In considering what we can work on, it may make sense for us to set as a goal to address this unhealthy negative emotion of jealousy and move toward disappointment when you see him looking at her. (Criterion 1, Component A) This might then prevent you from grilling and nagging him. (Criterion 1, Component B) Are we in agreement that our first goal will be to replace the jealousy with disappointment when you see him looking at her? (Criterion 2)

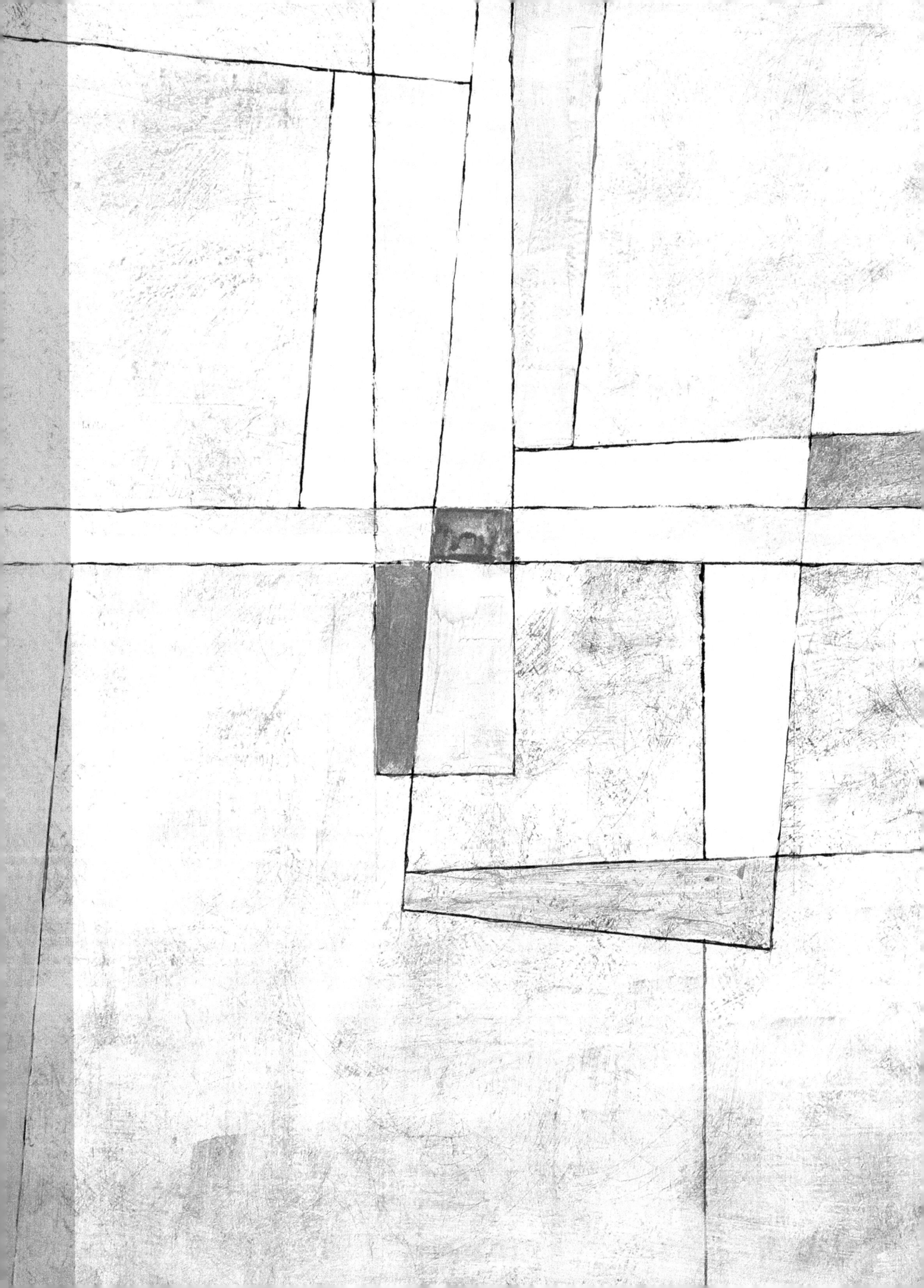

Clarifying Inferences From Irrational Beliefs

Preparations for Exercise 4

1. Read the instructions in Chapter 2.

2. Download the Deliberate Practice Reaction Form and the Deliberate Practice Diary Form at https://www.apa.org/pubs/books/deliberate-practice-rational-emotive-behavior-therapy (see the "Clinician and Practitioner Resources" tab; also available in Appendixes A and B, respectively).

Skill Description

Skill Difficulty Level: Beginner

Disputing irrational beliefs is one of the primary clinical interventions at the core of rational emotive behavior therapy (REBT). It involves collaboratively and directly challenging clients' irrational beliefs. An obstacle often seen clinically is that clients often present with both inferences (e.g., "He doesn't like me") and irrational evaluative beliefs (e.g., "It is awful that he doesn't like me") or an irrational, demanding belief (e.g., "He must like me"). REBT uses the term *inferences* to reflect what some other cognitive behavioral theories call cognitive errors, cognitive distortions, or negative automatic thoughts. These thoughts are ideas about the self, others, or the world that people infer from the perceptions that they have of the world. The inferences reflect the client's thought on what the world is. REBT defines *irrational beliefs* as demands, excessive negative evaluations of events (e.g., awfulizing, catastrophizing), global evaluation of human and life worth (of the self, others, or the world), or statements about one's endurance or frustration intolerance (DiGiuseppe et al., 2014). An important distinction between the inferences and the evaluative beliefs is reflected in how some cognitive behavior therapy

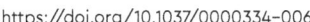
https://doi.org/10.1037/0000334-006

Deliberate Practice in Rational Emotive Behavior Therapy, by M. D. Terjesen, K. A. Doyle, R. A. DiGiuseppe, A. Vaz, and T. Rousmaniere

(CBT) theories refer to the inferences as automatic thoughts because they are experienced spontaneously in the person's stream of consciousness and require no effort to pop into one's head. Irrational beliefs are evaluative beliefs and are more tacit cognitions. That is, people are not always aware they have them. Thus, they might first experience inferences and the irrational beliefs mixed in with the inferences.

Cognitive restructuring often focuses on changing both thoughts and beliefs. Still, REBT practitioners stress the importance of changing irrational beliefs, which are demands or evaluative beliefs that are at the core of emotional and behavioral change. As clients can intertwine their inferences with their irrational beliefs, the goal of this exercise is to help clinicians collaborate with clients to understand the difference between inferences and irrational beliefs.

This skill requires the clinician to consider what thoughts and beliefs the client presents and differentiate inferences from irrational beliefs. Again, irrational beliefs come in two categories. The first is imperative demands that things should be a certain way. Second, an irrational belief can be an exaggerated evaluation of the event, a person (the self or another), or of the person's ability to tolerate the event. This skill requires the clinician to help the client (a) understand the differences between their inferences and their irrational beliefs and that their disturbance (i.e., emotional and/or behavioral) derives primarily from irrational beliefs and (b) agree to target the demanding or evaluative beliefs for change.

Special Considerations for Exercise 4

Please note that for the beginner difficulty client statements, the inference(s) and irrational belief(s) are presented directly in the client statements. The intermediate difficulty client statements have a direct inference stated, but the evaluative or demanding irrational beliefs are implied. Finally, for the advanced difficulty client statements, both the inference and the evaluative and demanding beliefs are implied. The goal is for the reader to build on the skills because clients do not always present their inferences and irrational beliefs clearly and directly.

SKILL CRITERIA FOR EXERCISE 4

1. Reflect the initial inferential thoughts presented by the client.
2. Reflect the initial irrational beliefs presented by the client.
3. Offer psychoeducation to differentiate inferences from irrational beliefs.
4. Check with the client to see whether they understand that the irrational demand or evaluative irrational belief will be the target for change.

Examples of Therapists Clarifying Inferences From Irrational Beliefs

Example 1

CLIENT: [*angry*] My colleagues don't respect me and my effort in building our company. I get so angry at them for not doing their work and even more for the lack of respect. They should treat me like they want to be treated.

THERAPIST: I hear two related but distinct thoughts. The first thought is that "they don't respect you and you have earned their respect." That thought might or might not be true. We can examine the accuracy of that inference later. (Criterion 1) The second thought is, "They should respect me." It reflects an irrational demand belief about their behavior. (Criterion 2) Emotional and behavioral difficulties are caused more by irrational beliefs. That is, demanding beliefs are illogical, self-defeating in that they block us from achieving our goals, and they are not consistent with what we know to be true. That belief sounds like it is "they **should** treat me with respect." Inferences and demanding beliefs are different based on what I just described. We believe that this belief creates most of your anger. (Criterion 3) Although it sounds like you have both thoughts, do you understand that we will try to change the irrational belief that your colleagues **should** respect you? (Criterion 4)

Example 2

CLIENT: [*anxious*] I had the first day of theater rehearsal, and all of a sudden I felt sick. I couldn't breathe. I was sweating. And all my thoughts concerned how I could avoid going. This year is a musical, and I was so anxious about the idea that other students who are trying out will make fun of me. Theater means so much to me, and if they make fun of me, I don't even know what I would do; I'd probably quit theater, which I love.

THERAPIST: It sounds like you were feeling anxious and experienced a few related but separate ideas in your head. It sounds like the initial thought was that the other students would make fun of you. (Criterion 1) Although that might be true, we can examine the accuracy of that thought later. And while you didn't state it, the second idea that I hear is, "**If** they did make fun of me, that would be awful." This idea is an irrational evaluation of the situation. (Criterion 2) Unlike the inference, which might or might not be accurate, irrational evaluative ideas are not helpful, not consistent with reality, and do not make sense. There is a difference between that inference "they will make fun of me" and the evaluative belief "it would be awful if they made fun of me." (Criterion 3) Suppose our goal is to help you feel concerned rather than anxious about being made fun of and to have you still participate in theater. What do you think about our changing the evaluative belief that "it would be awful to be made fun of" that creates the anxiety? Could we focus on that for change? (Criterion 4)

Example 3

CLIENT: [*depressed*] No matter how hard I try or how dedicated I am to someone in a relationship, it always fails or doesn't work out. Clearly, something I am doing or something about me turns people off. I will never be in a successful relationship. I feel so depressed when I see everyone around me having happy relationships, yet I cannot have one. Sometimes I break down and cry. I can't even have a relationship that lasts more than 3 months.

THERAPIST: What you are describing sounds like depression, and I hear you have a few types of thoughts that go with it. You infer that something you are doing or something about you is the reason you are not in a relationship. (Criterion 1) That thought might be accurate or inaccurate, and we can examine the accuracy of that thought together. You make another inference that you will never be in a relationship. (Criterion 1) Again, that may be true, but those inferences are one type of thought. The second type of thought I hear from you is considered more of an irrational belief. It is a global evaluation of yourself that you are a complete loser because you cannot maintain a relationship. This irrational belief differs from the inferences and might have a greater impact on your feelings. This irrational belief is not consistent with reality, doesn't help you feel better, and doesn't make sense. (Criterion 2) This irrational belief differs from the inferences and might have a greater impact on your emotions. (Criterion 3) If you want to feel sad rather than depressed and be better able to pursue relationships, do you think it would be more helpful to change the global, negative self-evaluative belief "I am a loser"? (Criterion 4)

INSTRUCTIONS FOR EXERCISE 4

Step 1: Role-Play and Feedback

- The client says the first beginner client statement. The therapist **improvises** a response based on the skill criteria.
- The trainer (or if not available, the client) provides **brief** feedback based on the skill criteria.
- The client then repeats the same statement, and the therapist again improvises a response. The trainer (or client) again provides brief feedback.

Step 2: Repeat

- Repeat Step 1 for all the statements **in the current difficulty level** (beginner, intermediate, or advanced).

Step 3: Assess and Adjust Difficulty

- The therapist completes the Deliberate Practice Reaction Form (see Appendix A) and decides whether to make the exercise easier or harder or to repeat the same difficulty level.

Step 4: Repeat for Approximately 15 Minutes

- Repeat Steps 1 to 3 for at least 15 minutes.
- The trainees then switch therapist and client roles and start over.

> **Now it's your turn! Follow Steps 1 and 2 from the instructions.**

Remember: The goal of the role-play is for trainees to practice improvising responses to the client statements in a manner that (a) uses the skill criteria and (b) feels authentic for the trainee. **Example therapist responses for each client statement are provided at the end of this exercise. Trainees should attempt to improvise their own responses before reading the example responses.**

BEGINNER-LEVEL CLIENT STATEMENTS FOR EXERCISE 4
Beginner Client Statement 1
[Angry] This is the third time in a week I couldn't find something. I give very clear directions to the office administrator, and he never does it correctly. He doesn't seem to care about his job. I get so angry as he gets paid a decent salary and really should do what he is paid to do.
Beginner Client Statement 2
[Depressed] The pandemic has led us to cancel many family plans. I think some people use this pandemic as an excuse not to get together, and they really don't seem to care about me. What kind of mother am I that they don't care enough to visit me? I must be a pretty bad person for people not to want to spend time with me. I am so depressed about this.
Beginner Client Statement 3
[Guilty] I lied to my boss. She asked me if I had followed the memo and checked the reports before they went out. I said yes when I hadn't really done it. Anyone else would have either checked the reports or have been honest about it. I feel so guilty because this is going to come back and be a problem at some point. I should have done the right thing.
Beginner Client Statement 4
[Anxious] We are moving in the middle of the school year, and I am worried that my son will have difficulty adjusting to school and making friends. He has always struggled socially and academically, and I feel like I am setting him up for failure. What if it is a mistake? That would just be the worst thing that could happen to him, as it would set him back for years, and I wouldn't be able to stand it.
Beginner Client Statement 5
[Jealous] My partner seems to be spending more and more time with his work colleagues than with me. I do not know for certain, but I hear his conference calls with one female colleague, and they border on flirtatious. I could see him leaving me for her. There are times I want to call them both out on their behavior, but I refrain. But honestly, these thoughts stick with me for hours. He shouldn't act this way and instead should focus on our relationship.

 Assess and adjust the difficulty before moving to the next difficulty level (see Step 3 in the exercise instructions).

INTERMEDIATE-LEVEL CLIENT STATEMENTS FOR EXERCISE 4
Intermediate Client Statement 1
[Angry] I got so angry with my ex-wife. When she sends my son over for visitation, she sends him with a bag of food to eat. It is like she does not think I am competent to feed him. She wants him to see me as an irresponsible and a bad dad. How can she do such a thing to me?
Intermediate Client Statement 2
[Depressed] I have been depressed about work. I have so many projects that are due at work. I know that I can't complete them all, let alone do them well. People are going to notice and think I am irresponsible. They will think I'm a loser. What does that mean about me?
Intermediate Client Statement 3
[Guilty] This week was the anniversary of my brother's death. I think about all the troubles he had, being disabled, and I think I could have been a better brother. I could have helped him more. I just didn't do enough to help him. Did I do right by him?
Intermediate Client Statement 4
[Anxious] Winter is here, and I always feel more anxious in winter. There are storms, and it's cold. I question whether I can cope with it. So many terrible things can happen, it is cold, you can't go out, and things can happen to your house. It is just so hard to make it through the winter.
Intermediate Client Statement 5
[Jealous] My partner talks a lot about this person at work. She seems to really admire him and thinks he is so talented. When she talks about him, I feel jealous, like she might be more attracted to him than she is to me. Could I survive it if she left me for him?

 Assess and adjust the difficulty before moving to the next difficulty level (see Step 3 in the exercise instructions).

ADVANCED-LEVEL CLIENT STATEMENTS FOR EXERCISE 4
Advanced Client Statement 1
[Angry] I was on the bus the other evening, and it has been made very clear that people are to wear masks on public transportation due to the pandemic. Sitting across from me is a guy, no mask on, nonchalantly checking his phone. I was enraged and could not stop thinking about him. He clearly doesn't care about anyone but himself. How could he act this way?
Advanced Client Statement 2
[Depressed] My world is getting smaller. No one calls me anymore because they think I'm boring. This is so depressing. What if they're right? That would not be saying anything great about me.
Advanced Client Statement 3
[Guilty] I haven't finished this work project that was due months ago. I want to get it done, but it keeps getting pushed to the bottom of the list, which means it's never going to get completed. I feel so bad that others are waiting on me. When did I become "that" person?
Advanced Client Statement 4
[Anxious] I haven't gone to the doctor since way before COVID hit. I know when I go, they're going to find something wrong with me. The idea of that makes me cringe, and I keep putting off making the appointment.
Advanced Client Statement 5
[Jealous] She's not paying as much attention to me as she used to, clearly because she's not into me anymore. She pays more attention to other guys. I really want this relationship, but she seems to be more interested in other guys. What's wrong with me?

 Assess and adjust the difficulty here (see Step 3 in the exercise instructions). If appropriate, follow the instructions to make the exercise even more challenging (see Appendix A).

Example Therapist Responses: Clarifying Inferences From Irrational Beliefs

Remember: Trainees should attempt to improvise their own responses before reading the example responses. **Do not read the following responses verbatim unless you are having trouble coming up with your own responses!**

EXAMPLE RESPONSES TO BEGINNER-LEVEL CLIENT STATEMENTS FOR EXERCISE 4
Example Response to Beginner Client Statement 1
I hear three thoughts here. First, he "never does it correctly" and, second, "He doesn't care about his job." (Criterion 1) Both are inferences you draw for the situation, and we can see whether they are accurate. The third thought I hear you saying is that he should do his job. (Criterion 2) This idea can be a demand about his behavior. Unlike the two inferences, "should" beliefs are irrational because they are not helpful, not in line with reality as he did what he did, and that they do not make sense. (Criterion 3) We want to distinguish between the first two inferences ("He doesn't care, and he never does it correctly") and the irrational, demanding belief ("He should do it correctly"). (Criterion 3) Do you think it would be better to change the irrational, demanding belief of "He should do it correctly" that creates your anger? (Criterion 4)
Example Response to Beginner Client Statement 2
I hear an inference that they don't care about you. (Criterion 1) We can investigate whether that thought is accurate or not. However, you have a second belief, "I'm a pretty bad person." (Criterion 2) This belief is referred to as an irrational global evaluation of yourself. Here you are evaluating your worth, which we will show is inaccurate, not helpful, and nonsensical. That first inference ("They don't care about me") is different from the global self-evaluative belief ("I am a pretty bad person"). And it is this type of idea that contributes more to your depression. (Criterion 3) As we work to change your experience of depression, do you think it would be more helpful to focus on changing the irrational evaluative belief rather than the inference because the inference, unfortunately, could be accurate? (Criterion 4)
Example Response to Beginner Client Statement 3
Your guilt occurred when you experienced two related but distinct types of ideas. The first group of thoughts are inferences about what happened. These include the ideas that first, anyone else would have checked; second, others would have been honest about it; and third, this will become a problem at some point. While those ideas might be true, you are making inferences or conclusions that might not come true. (Criterion 1) The second type of idea you had is "I should have done the right thing." This is a demand on your behavior. (Criterion 2) Unlike the inference, which might or might not be accurate, these demanding beliefs are irrational because they are not helpful toward your goals, are not consistent with reality, and aren't logical. There is a difference between these inferences and demanding beliefs. (Criterion 3) If our goal is to get you to regret your behavior, does it make sense to change the demands that led to your feeling of guilt? (Criterion 4)

Example Response to Beginner Client Statement 4

It sounds like you feel anxious when you have a few thoughts about the move and its potential impact on your son. The first thought is that you are setting him up for failure and he will have difficulty adjusting. (Criterion 1) We don't know if that inference or conclusion is correct, and we can examine the likelihood that those thoughts are true. The second idea that I hear is that if he does have difficulty adjusting, it would be the worst and you couldn't stand seeing him struggling. (Criterion 2) These are irrational evaluative beliefs concerning the potential situation. Unlike the inference, which may or may not be accurate, the irrational beliefs are not helpful in achieving your goal. They are not true, and it does not make sense to think you could not stand this or that it would be the worst. This is an important distinction between that first inference and the evaluative belief. (Criterion 3) If our goal is to get you to feel concerned about the move and its impact on your son, do you think it best that we change the evaluative beliefs of "I couldn't stand it" and "it would be the worst thing for him" that creates the anxiety? (Criterion 4)

Example Response to Beginner Client Statement 5

If changing your jealousy is the main goal, it would be important to explore the truth of these thoughts that lead to jealousy. I hear some inferences here. First, he spends more time with work colleagues. Second, he flirts with one of them. And third he could leave you. Those thoughts, while upsetting, might be true or might be untrue. (Criterion 1) We can examine the accuracy of those thoughts. The second idea that I hear is that he should not act this way. (Criterion 2) This idea is a demand of his behavior. This demanding belief is considered irrational because it won't help you work toward your goals. It is not consistent with reality—he can act differently, and it is not logical to believe that because you want him not to act this way, that he must not. We want to consider the difference between that first set of three inferences ("He spends more time with work, is flirtatious, and could leave me") and the demanding belief ("He shouldn't act this way"). (Criterion 3) If our goal is to change your jealousy, what is your reaction to our initially focusing on changing the demanding belief that creates your jealousy? (Criterion 4)

EXAMPLE RESPONSES TO INTERMEDIATE-LEVEL CLIENT STATEMENTS FOR EXERCISE 4

Example Response to Intermediate Client Statement 1

You have identified several thoughts in your head when you become angry at her. The first two are inferences you draw because she sends your son with food. You think that she does not see you as competent and wants your son to see you the same way. (Criterion 1) Those are ideas you infer from her behavior, and we could examine them to see if they are true. It sounds like you have another idea behind your questions, "How could she do this?" That may reflect a belief that "she must not do things like question my competence or make me look bad in front of our son." (Criterion 2) This second type of belief we call demandingness. Here you demand that she should not do this behavior. This rigidly held idea is not accurate, not helpful, and is different from that initial thought you had that she does not see you as competent. (Criterion 3) Do you agree that it is best to target the demanding beliefs that are associated with your anger? (Criterion 4)

Example Response to Intermediate Client Statement 2

When you talk about your depression, you associate it with several thoughts. First, you infer that you cannot get your jobs done or do them well and other people will perceive you as an irresponsible loser. (Criterion 1) These things could happen, but you could be overestimating their likelihood. It sounds like you think that if they were true, you would be an irresponsible loser. (Criterion 2) Such an irrational, global, and negative self-evaluation is a different type of belief. It focuses only on your errors and equates who you are and your worth based on those failings. (Criterion 3) Do you see the value of separating those initial thoughts and evaluative beliefs and how focusing on your self-evaluations could be more helpful in changing your depression to sadness? (Criteria 4)

Example Response to Intermediate Client Statement 3

Your guilt about your brother seems linked to several thoughts. You think that you did not help him enough with his disability. (Criterion 1) This thought is an inference or conclusion you made from what happened. It is hard to evaluate whether it is true or not because who is to say how much was enough. But you could also have an additional belief, such as "Whatever I did for my brother, I should have done more." (Criterion 2) While the first thought, "I did not do enough," is an inference, the idea that "I should have done more" represents a demand on what should have happened. The thought I did not do enough and the belief that you should have done more are different. (Criterion 3) Do you agree that the second "should" belief is more important in causing your guilt and, as a result, we may want to target it initially for change? (Criterion 4)

Example Response to Intermediate Client Statement 4

Your anxiety about the season seems related to several different thoughts in your head. There will be storms, snow, and lots of things to keep you in, and there are things that can damage your house. (Criterion 1) All these ideas are present and could be true. Perhaps you are having another idea that is of a different type. You seem to think that all the problems of winter are things that you cannot endure. (Criterion 2) This is an irrational belief about your strength and endurance. (Criteria 3) The ideas about what could happen differ from your perceived strength to deal with them. (Criterion 3) Do you see that your irrational evaluation of your strength to handle the winter is more of the problem than thoughts about what could happen, and it would be more helpful to target this idea for change? (Criterion 4)

Example Response to Intermediate Client Statement 5

You mentioned two sets of thoughts about her behavior that connect to your jealousy. The first set are ideas you infer from her behavior. You think that she admires the guy at work, thinks he is talented, and she might be more attracted to him than she is to you. (Criterion 1) These ideas help trigger the jealousy, and they might or might not be true. However, it sounds like you think you can't stand it if those ideas were true. (Criterion 2) Although the first group of thoughts are inferences that may be incorrect, the belief that you can't stand this is more evaluative and irrational in nature. (Criterion 3) Do you see how the idea that you could not tolerate it if these inferences were true is more related to your jealousy, and it would be better to target that belief than the thought that she is attracted to the other guy? (Criterion 4)

**EXAMPLE RESPONSES TO ADVANCED-LEVEL
CLIENT STATEMENTS FOR EXERCISE 4**

Example Response to Advanced Client Statement 1

You appear to be drawing a conclusion or an inference that this guy doesn't care about the rules or other people. (Criterion 1) You might be right about this conclusion, but you could also be wrong. However, as you discuss being enraged, you also appear shocked by what he has done. Perhaps this expresses the demand that he should respect the rules and the safety of others. (Criterion 2) The problem here is that he was not doing so, and you got yourself enraged and ruminated about it, while he sat maskless! There is an important distinction between your inference and that demand in how much they contribute to your anger. (Criterion 3) If your goal is not to get enraged, might it make sense first to address your demands concerning how he should be acting? (Criterion 4)

Example Response to Advanced Client Statement 2

You're telling me that because people are not calling you anymore, your world is getting smaller, and people think you're boring. (Criterion 1) We could examine these inferences, and if they are inaccurate, you will be relieved. However, if they are accurate, you won't be helped. On the other hand, I'm hearing a message that if people thought you were boring, it would mean something bad about you as a person, such as that you're inadequate. (Criterion 2) It sounds like you have the inferences and the evaluation of your self-worth if your inferences are true. (Criterion 3) If your goal is to not feel depressed about your situation, can you see why it makes more sense to work on your evaluation of your worth as a person? (Criterion 4)

Example Response to Advanced Client Statement 3

I hear you drawing the conclusion that the project will never get done, (Criterion 1) something we call an inference. Yet I also hear that you might be feeling guilty because you're demanding that you should have finished the project, and because you didn't, you're evaluating yourself globally as a failure. (Criterion 2) Given that your demand and global self-rating are contributing more to your guilt, which is not helping you complete the project, (Criterion 3) do you think that it would be best to address your demandingness and ratings of worth evaluation? (Criterion 4)

Example Response to Advanced Client Statement 4

It sounds like your anxiety is linked to the conclusion you're making that the doctor will find something wrong with you, (Criterion 1) which may or may not occur, resulting in your avoiding making the appointment. However, when you "cringe," might you have some catastrophizing beliefs and frustration intolerance about the possibility of something being wrong with you? (Criterion 2) There is a difference between the conclusion that something is wrong with you and the evaluative belief that it would be catastrophic and intolerable. (Criterion 3) Might it be more helpful to start challenging the catastrophizing and frustration intolerance to help you push through and make the appointment, given that your conclusion that the doctor will find something wrong may not be accurate? (Criterion 4)

Example Response to Advanced Client Statement 5

This inference that she is not into you anymore (Criterion 1) is something we could examine to see whether it is accurate, but we might never get the real answer. On the other hand, I also hear in your words ideas like she should be paying more attention to you, and because she's not, there's something globally wrong with you, like you're worthless or inadequate as a person. We would describe those as irrational beliefs. (Criterion 2) There is a difference between your inference and your irrational beliefs. The inference can be factually true or false. But the demand and global self-downing irrational beliefs do not help you cope emotionally in this situation. (Criterion 3) Because your irrational beliefs create that jealousy, do you agree that we work on those beliefs first and then perhaps revisit your inference later? (Criterion 4)

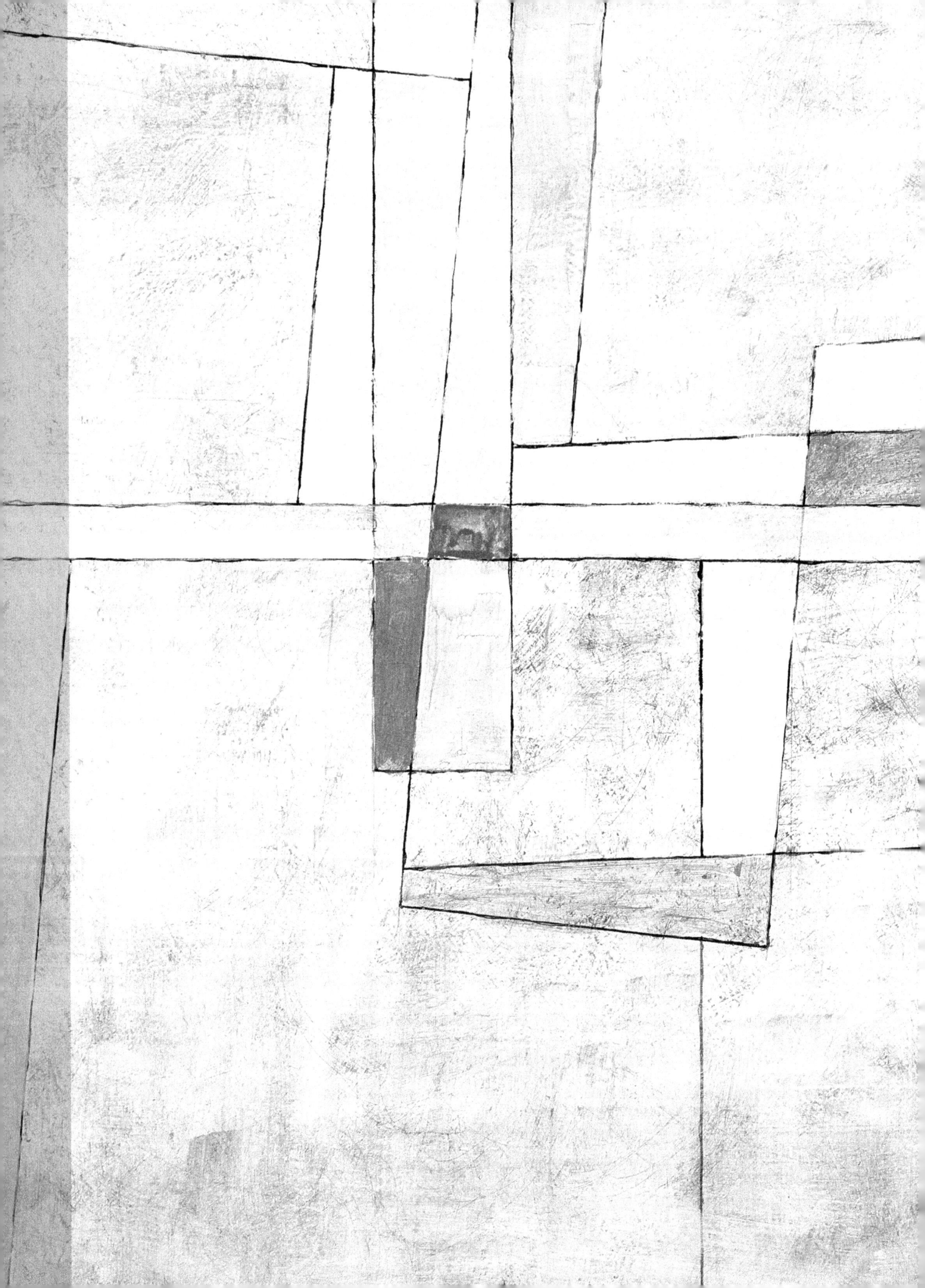

Assessing Irrational Beliefs About the Activating Event

Preparations for Exercise 5

1. Read the instructions in Chapter 2.

2. Download the Deliberate Practice Reaction Form and the Deliberate Practice Diary Form at https://www.apa.org/pubs/books/deliberate-practice-rational-emotive-behavior-therapy (see the "Clinician and Practitioner Resources" tab; also available in Appendixes A and B, respectively).

Skill Description

Skill Difficulty Level: Intermediate

In the prior exercise, we worked on having clients learn the differences between automatic thoughts or inferences and irrational beliefs. A clinical intervention that is among the most integral to the process of rational emotive behavior therapy (REBT) is to assess and identify accurately the specific irrational belief(s) the client has about the activating event (the A in the ABC model from Exercise 1) or situation. REBT theory holds that these beliefs are often what lead to the emotional and behavioral consequence(s) (Cs) that clients come to therapy to change. Subsequent clinical skills within REBT such as the prioritization of which irrational belief to focus on (Exercise 6), connection of this irrational belief to the consequence (Exercise 7), disputation of these irrational beliefs (Exercises 8–10), and eventually changing these irrational beliefs to rational alternatives (Exercise 11) are much more difficult to do without a thorough assessment of the irrational belief. Irrational beliefs are conceptualized to consist of demands as well as derivatives (awfulizing, frustration intolerance, ratings of worth) of the demand. These beliefs are discussed with clients during the initial psychoeducation of REBT (Exercises 1 and 2).

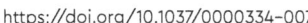

https://doi.org/10.1037/0000334-007

Deliberate Practice in Rational Emotive Behavior Therapy, by M. D. Terjesen, K. A. Doyle, R. A. DiGiuseppe, A. Vaz, and T. Rousmaniere

REBT theory proposes that the primary belief is a demand that may have an accompanying derivative(s) about activating events, and it is recommended that clinicians assess the presence of all the irrational beliefs that lead to unhealthy negative emotions and/or maladaptive behaviors and examine how those beliefs may differ from more healthy, rational ones. That is, assess the belief and the dysfunctionality of it and differentiate it from the rational beliefs about these situations.

Special Considerations for Performing This Exercise

Please note that the first five beginner-level statements have the client explicitly state their irrational belief(s), while the next five intermediate-level statements include one evident irrational belief and another one that is inferred, and finally the last five advanced-level statements do not explicitly state any irrational beliefs from the client.

To best understand and conceptualize the specific irrational beliefs of each activating event, it is important that trainees have a strong understanding of the REBT conceptualization of emotions. For a more advanced review, refer to Dryden, David, and Ellis (2010). For the five emotions that the client experiences as a result of these activating events, consider the irrational beliefs that are typically associated with each emotion. More specifically, for anger, the common irrational beliefs are demandingness and other-downing. With depression, one often finds beliefs of demandingness and self-condemnation. Anxiety is typically associated with irrational beliefs of demandingness and awfulizing, but frustration intolerance is also commonly present. With guilt as the primary emotion, the irrational beliefs present are often demandingness and self-ratings. For jealousy, the irrational beliefs are typically demandingness and ratings of worth. It is important to remember that these are only guidelines and that when working with clients, they can hold several of the four irrational beliefs. It is important to develop hypotheses based on their unhealthy negative emotions or maladaptive behaviors, but remember to offer them to the client and get feedback. This format aims to help you organically enhance your skills in assessing beliefs that your clients hold.

SKILL CRITERIA FOR EXERCISE 5

1. Propose the existence of a demand as well as any derivative evaluative irrational beliefs.
2. Distinguish these demands and evaluative irrational beliefs and their consequences from those of the rational beliefs.

Examples of Therapists Assessing Irrational Beliefs About the Activating Event

Example 1

CLIENT: [*angry*] I get so angry when people keep pushing me to change my schedule to accommodate theirs. It's wrong, and they shouldn't do it. I really can't deal with this much longer. It drives me nuts and I ruminate about it, lose sleep from it, and then hold it against them, which isn't good for me personally or professionally.

THERAPIST: It sounds like when you feel anger, you have two beliefs here. One is a demand that they shouldn't do that, and the other is more of a frustration intolerance belief that you can't deal with it. Often with anger, the demanding belief is the strongest one that causes greater negative consequences. (Criterion 1) The alternative to these irrational beliefs is more rational ones that would lead you to experience a more healthy emotion, such as annoyance, when people push you to change your schedule. Here, instead of believing that demand that people shouldn't do that, the rational alternative would be "I really would like or prefer that they not do this, but there is no reason that they must do what I want them to" and instead of believing that you can't deal with it, the rational alternative would be "I don't like this, but I can stand or deal with it." (Criterion 2)

Example 2

CLIENT: [*anxious*] I am so worried about getting all my work done. I have taken on more responsibilities than one could expect to manage and really shouldn't have. I know I am going to mess up on something and end up avoiding doing it. My colleague who I am working with will be upset at me and not want to work with me again, and that would be the worst.

THERAPIST: Typically, when people are anxious like you seem to be, there are a couple of different beliefs that may lead to that feeling. Based on what you said, one may be more of a demand that you shouldn't have taken on all those responsibilities, and the other is more of an awfulizing belief when you say that it would be the worst if your colleague was upset with you. This demand is likely the original and perhaps the stronger of the two beliefs and may contribute to your feelings of anxiety and avoidance of doing the work. (Criterion 1) Alternatively, we can work on more rational beliefs about this situation that would allow you to experience a healthier negative emotion such as concern when you think about your work responsibilities. Perhaps instead of believing the demand that "I shouldn't have taken on all these responsibilities," the rational alternative would be "I really wish that I had not done so, but I annoyingly did and there's nothing that says I should not have." Instead of believing that it would be the worst if your colleague was upset with you, the rational alternative would be "It would be bad, but not terrible or awful if my colleague was upset with me." (Criterion 2)

Example 3

CLIENT: [*depressed*] I feel so depressed and hopeless. Once we broke up, my social circle has gotten much smaller. People seem to have chosen to remain friends with my ex-partner rather than me. I should not have made the mistake of leaving my friends behind and dedicating my social life to making my ex-partner happy. The fact that people have all left me just shows what a dumb decision that was and how truly unlikeable and worthless I am.

THERAPIST: Your feelings of depression may come from a few different beliefs that you have about your situation. I hear two primary ones: one, that you shouldn't have made the friend decisions that you did and, two, because people left you, that means you are worthless. That initial demand belief about your decision may contribute more strongly to your feelings of depression and then set the stage for the second worthless belief. (Criterion 1) What may be helpful is for us to develop more rational beliefs about this situation, which would lead to a more healthy negative emotion, such as sadness. If we are able to change the demand belief that "I shouldn't have made the friend decisions that I did" to a more rational alternative of "I really wish I had made different decisions, but there's no reason I absolutely must have," we may be able to move toward that healthier negative emotion of sadness. Further, instead of believing that "I am worthless because of my decisions and the size of my friends circle," the rational alternative would be "My worth or value does not depend on the decisions I make, whether good or bad" and that too may help us work towards healthier goals. (Criterion 2)

INSTRUCTIONS FOR EXERCISE 5

Step 1: Role-Play and Feedback

- The client says the first beginner client statement. The therapist **improvises** a response based on the skill criteria.
- The trainer (or if not available, the client) provides **brief** feedback based on the skill criteria.
- The client then repeats the same statement, and the therapist again improvises a response. The trainer (or client) again provides brief feedback.

Step 2: Repeat

- Repeat Step 1 for all the statements **in the current difficulty level** (beginner, intermediate, or advanced).

Step 3: Assess and Adjust Difficulty

- The therapist completes the Deliberate Practice Reaction Form (see Appendix A) and decides whether to make the exercise easier or harder or to repeat the same difficulty level.

Step 4: Repeat for Approximately 15 Minutes

- Repeat Steps 1 to 3 for at least 15 minutes.
- The trainees then switch therapist and client roles and start over.

> **Now it's your turn! Follow Steps 1 and 2 from the instructions.**

Remember: The goal of the role-play is for trainees to practice improvising responses to the client statements in a manner that (a) uses the skill criteria and (b) feels authentic for the trainee. **Example therapist responses for each client statement are provided at the end of this exercise. Trainees should attempt to improvise their own responses before reading the example responses.**

BEGINNER-LEVEL CLIENT STATEMENTS FOR EXERCISE 5
Beginner Client Statement 1
[Angry] Every time I get what my parents consider to be a bad grade, they come into my room and take away all my technology. They never ask my side of the story, and I get so angry at them. They should leave my stuff alone. They do this all the time, and I end up flipping out. I really can't stand it.
Beginner Client Statement 2
[Depressed] I see the pathway that my adult son is taking in life, and frankly it saddens me and I get depressed about it. He is always going to struggle, and it really is my fault. I am to blame and am not only a bad parent but a bad person. I should have done a better job as a parent. I refused to let him learn how to handle disappointment, always covered for him, and probably was overprotective of him.
Beginner Client Statement 3
[Guilty] I keep on agreeing to take on assignments that are due in 6 months when I have already unofficially accepted a job with a new company in 4 months. This will totally screw them. I feel so guilty—they are so nice to me, and I should have the courage to tell them the truth. The idea that these friends and colleagues will think poorly about me after I leave is too difficult to deal with.
Beginner Client Statement 4
[Anxious] My son and daughter-in-law will be moving in with me for the next 6 months while their home is being renovated. I am so anxious that this will be the end of any kind of relationship that we have. They always fight and make my home very uncomfortable. They should have rented a place. The next 6 months will truly be the worst.
Beginner Client Statement 5
[Jealous] We both applied for the same clinical training position, and it went to a person that I really do not respect. I think she had an "in" with the director. I have better credentials than her, and I should at least have been offered an interview. I cannot handle this level of unfairness.

🔘 **Assess and adjust the difficulty before moving to the next difficulty level (see Step 3 in the exercise instructions).**

INTERMEDIATE-LEVEL CLIENT STATEMENTS FOR EXERCISE 5
Intermediate Client Statement 1
[Angry] This is the third time my son has gotten a traffic violation, and it keeps driving up our insurance. No matter how many times we tell him, he just doesn't listen. It's like he doesn't even care about the fact that we have to pay more now.
Intermediate Client Statement 2
[Depressed] It is now coming up on a year since I had a full-time job. My partner continues to tell me just to apply to anything, but why would anyone want to hire someone who has huge gaps in their employment history? It really says something about me that no one will hire me.
Intermediate Client Statement 3
[Guilty] I definitely am the weak link in our partnership at work. I use any excuse to do less than my partner, because I know they will end up doing it anyway. I feel so bad about this.
Intermediate Client Statement 4
[Anxious] This presentation is now taking on a whole new focus with Saul having announced his retirement from the firm. I know they will be looking to see who can fill his shoes and, while I think I have a pretty good track record, those worry butterflies we have spoken about are taking over and causing me considerable stress.
Intermediate Client Statement 5
[Jealous] As we were celebrating my 1-year anniversary of being in this position, my former boss came back. This was to be my day, my moment, and sure enough, everyone is happy to see him, coming over and acting like he is still the boss and getting all the attention.

 Assess and adjust the difficulty before moving to the next difficulty level (see Step 3 in the exercise instructions).

ADVANCED-LEVEL CLIENT STATEMENTS FOR EXERCISE 5
Advanced Client Statement 1
[Angry] I find that I am getting more and more angry at my neighbors in my building. They are young and clearly don't realize what it's like to live in a New York City building. They're loud, let their doors slam, and have parties until all hours of the night. Recently, I've gotten into verbal altercations with some of them, which of course I am not proud of. I mean, really, what are these people thinking?
Advanced Client Statement 2
[Depressed] The anniversary of my husband's death is coming up soon and it's always this time of year that I start to isolate myself. Waves of depression come on, I cry a lot, and ruminate about how young he was and the way he died.
Advanced Client Statement 3
[Guilty] I have a lot of guilt about avoiding calling a colleague of mine who recently lost his wife. I think about calling, and then I don't because I don't want to hear him cry. I feel so bad but that doesn't seem to get me to call. He's my friend and I'm not there for him.
Advanced Client Statement 4
[Anxious] I haven't gone to the doctor in many years because I'm really scared, maybe even anxious, about what they may find wrong. I've had so many people in my life die recently that it just freaks me out thinking about going and what could result, but I know it would be good to just get it over with.
Advanced Client Statement 5
[Jealous] I've noticed lately that my boyfriend is on the phone with one of his coworkers for extensive periods of time. Last night when I got home from work, he was on the phone with her for over an hour and didn't even acknowledge my presence. I can tell he really enjoys talking to her and he seems like a much happier person when he's talking with her. When he's with me he seems bored and disengaged.

 Assess and adjust the difficulty here (see Step 3 in the exercise instructions). If appropriate, follow the instructions to make the exercise even more challenging (see Appendix A).

Example Therapist Responses: Assessing Irrational Beliefs About the Activating Event

Remember: Trainees should attempt to improvise their own responses before reading the example responses. **Do not read the following responses verbatim unless you are having trouble coming up with your own responses!**

EXAMPLE RESPONSES TO BEGINNER-LEVEL CLIENT STATEMENTS FOR EXERCISE 5

Example Response to Beginner Client Statement 1

It sounds like when you feel angry at your parents that you have two beliefs. One is a demand that they should leave your stuff alone and probably that they should ask your side of the story and the other is more of a frustration intolerance belief that you can't deal with their behavior. Typically, with anger, the demanding belief is the strongest one that causes greater negative consequences, which in your case may be flipping out. (Criterion 1) To feel more frustrated at their behavior and perhaps not "flip out," we will want to develop an alternative or more rational belief to these irrational beliefs. Instead of demanding that they should leave your stuff alone, the rational alternative would be "I really want them to leave my stuff alone, but this is what they do and there is no reason that they must do what I want them to" and instead of believing that you can't stand it, the rational alternative would be "I don't like this, but they have done this before, and I stood it then. I can stand or deal with it." (Criterion 2)

Example Response to Beginner Client Statement 2

The depression that you describe may be the result of two beliefs that you have about yourself and the situation. The first is more of a rigidly held demand that you should have made better decisions, while the other is more of a ratings of worth where you equate your decisions with your worth or value as a person. These initial demands may give rise to the ratings of worth and are often the strongest one that causes the initial unhealthy emotional and behavioral consequences. (Criterion 1) We will work on changing these irrational beliefs to more rational ones, which in turn would lead you to experience a more healthy emotion such as sadness, regret, or disappointment. The rational alternative to that initial "should" or demand may be thinking "I really would have liked to make the right parenting decisions, but just because I want to have made the right ones, there is no reason that I should have" and instead of believing that you are a bad or worthless person because you possibly made bad decisions, the rational alternative would be: "I wish I didn't make some of the decisions I did, but that does not make me a bad or worthless person." (Criterion 2)

Example Response to Beginner Client Statement 3

You described feeling so guilty, and that feeling may come from two beliefs that you have about this situation. One is a demand that you should tell them the truth, and the other is more of a frustration intolerance belief that if they thought poorly about you, it would be too difficult to deal with it. Often with guilt, a demand, like you should have been telling the truth, is the initial belief that creates the feelings of guilt. (Criterion 1) If we want to change these feelings of guilt to more of a feeling of regret, we may wish to develop more rational or healthy alternative beliefs to these irrational ones. Working to change the guilt-inducing belief that "I should have told then the truth" to more of a healthier belief of "Perhaps I could have told them the truth, but believing that I should only causes me intense guilt. The truth is, I did not." As for the second belief, instead of believing that you can't deal with the possibility of them being upset with you, a more rational alternative would be: "If they do get upset with me, I won't like it, but I can stand or deal with it." (Criterion 2)

Example Response to Beginner Client Statement 4

Your anxiety about your son and daughter-in-law moving in with you most likely comes about from a few unhealthy or irrational beliefs. One is a demand that they should have rented another place, and the other belief is more of an awfulizing one, which is that the next 6 months will be the worst. Often with unhealthy negative emotions like anxiety, the demanding belief may be the first one we have, which then leads to the awfulizing thoughts. (Criterion 1) A rational belief would be a good, healthy alternative to the irrational ones and may help you feel a healthy level of concern about the next 6 months. Here, instead of that demanding belief that they should have rented a place, the rational alternative would be "I really wish that they had rented elsewhere, but there is no reason that they must do what I want them to" and instead of believing that the next 6 months will be the worst, the rational alternative would be "The next 6 months will probably be bad, but not as terrible as I believe." (Criterion 2)

Example Response to Beginner Client Statement 5

It sounds like when you feel jealous you have two beliefs here. One is a demand that you should have gotten an interview, and the other is that you can't deal with this level of unfairness. The demanding belief is typically considered to be the primary belief and the one that leads to unhealthy negative consequences, like feeling jealous. (Criterion 1) If we want to feel sad and regret and not be jealous about not getting the position, we will seek to develop an alternative rational belief to these irrational ones. Instead of believing that you should have gotten that position, a rational alternative would be "I really wish I had gotten that position and it may have been unfair, but there is no reason that they had to offer it to me." And instead of believing that you can't deal with the unfairness, the rational alternative would be "I don't like the possibility that this process was unfair, but I can stand or deal with it." (Criterion 2)

EXAMPLE RESPONSES TO INTERMEDIATE-LEVEL CLIENT STATEMENTS FOR EXERCISE 5

Example Response to Intermediate Client Statement 1

I hear some anger in what you are describing. Anger often comes from a demand and sometimes another type of belief. It sounds like you are thinking that he should just listen to you and that when he doesn't and gets a ticket that you can't stand it. (Criterion 1) To change your unhealthy feeling of anger, it may be helpful to replace those beliefs with healthier rational alternatives, such as "I really wish he would listen to me and be considerate, but there's no reason he must, and although I really don't like this, I can tolerate it." (Criterion 2)

Example Response to Intermediate Client Statement 2

It sounds like you're feeling depressed and that there are some beliefs that lead to that feeling as well as impact your lack of motivation to apply for these jobs. Sometimes, when people are depressed, they have beliefs like "I should be better," or, in your case, "I should be employed," and "because I am not, that just confirms that I am a complete loser." (Criterion 1) While no doubt it is frustrating to be unemployed for this long, I would like to propose that if you were truly able to believe something like "I really wish I was employed, but there's no law that says I must be, and just because I am not right now that does not make me a complete loser," you would feel more sadness instead of depression and also perhaps start applying for jobs. (Criterion 2)

Example Response to Intermediate Client Statement 3

Emotionally, what you are describing sounds like guilt. Very often, guilt is driven by beliefs that people have such as "I should hold up my end of the partnership and I'm a bad person that I don't." (Criterion 1) If we want to move away from the guilt toward regret, which is a healthy negative emotion, it may be good to change those "should" and self-condemnation beliefs to "I wish I had held up my end of the partnership, but there's no reason I absolutely must and my behavior is bad but that does not make me a bad person," which would probably result in strong regret. (Criterion 2)

Example Response to Intermediate Client Statement 4

It sounds like the stress that you are experiencing comes from some thoughts that you have about who they will put into Saul's position. This stress or worry may come from beliefs such as "They should offer me this position, and if they don't that would be the worst thing ever." (Criterion 1) If we work to change these unhealthy beliefs to healthier ones such as "I really want them to offer me this position, but if they don't, although that will be bad and disappointing, it really would not be the worst thing ever," I would predict that you would probably feel more concern than stress. (Criterion 2)

Example Response to Intermediate Client Statement 5

I imagine that event would be annoying to most people, but it sounds like you were experiencing some jealousy there. Jealousy often comes from beliefs such as "He shouldn't be getting all the attention, and it says something about me as a person that he is." (Criterion 1) The good thing is that if we are able to change these beliefs to healthier ones such as "I wish he wasn't getting all the attention, but there's nothing that says he must not, and if he does get attention and I don't, that doesn't define my worth as a person," you would probably feel more disappointment or annoyance. (Criterion 2)

EXAMPLE RESPONSES TO ADVANCED-LEVEL CLIENT STATEMENTS FOR EXERCISE 5

Example Response to Advanced Client Statement 1

I have a hypothesis about what you may be thinking when you feel anger toward your neighbors. I'm wondering if you are holding a rigid belief about how they should be courteous to their neighbors, and because they aren't, they're jerks. The first belief is a demand that is then followed by a derivative of other-condemnation or global ratings of others. (Criterion 1) To avoid future verbal altercations, which you mentioned you were not proud of, I think it would be worth considering changing your anger to a healthier negative emotion such as strong annoyance when they are not courteous. To do this, we will have to work on changing the irrational beliefs to healthier alternative rational ones. For example, "I really wish they would act more courteous toward their neighbors, but there is no reason that they must, and if they continue their behavior, it means they are flawed people but not total jerks." (Criterion 2)

Example Response to Advanced Client Statement 2

So this time of year tends to be more challenging than other times, and I'm sorry you're going through this. However, I do hear some possible beliefs that may be making a tough time for you even harder, one being a rigid demand that his death should not have happened at such a young age, and the other that it's awful that it did. (Criterion 1) If we work on changing this demand to a more flexible way of thinking, such as "I really wish this didn't happen to him, but unfortunately, there's no reason that unfortunate things must not happen," and change the other irrational belief to "It's so bad that this happened to him at such a young age, but it's not awful," perhaps when the anniversary comes up you would feel very strong sadness but not that depression. (Criterion 2)

Example Response to Advanced Client Statement 3

What I'm hearing you say when you report feeling guilt is an irrational, dogmatic demand you have of yourself that you should be calling your friend in his time of need. I also hear another irrational belief, sometimes referred to as a derivative of the demand, which is that because you have not called him, you are a bad person. (Criterion 1) If we want to work on moving you away from guilt and replace it with a healthier negative emotion about the current situation, such as regret, I think it would be helpful if we change that rigid demand you have of yourself to a more preferential desire. For example, "I really want to reach out to my friend, but there is no reason I absolutely must, and if I don't, that may be bad, but my behavior does not define me as a bad person." (Criterion 2)

Example Response to Advanced Client Statement 4

When I hear you say you feel anxious about going to the doctor because of what they may find, I hear several possible beliefs that may be contributing to this emotion. First, I wonder if you're thinking something like "I should go to the doctor," which we refer to as an irrational demand. I also hear that you may get news about your health that in your mind would be awful or terrible. Finally, I hear that you may be telling yourself that you couldn't stand to hear bad news, which is resulting in avoidance. (Criterion 1) For you to make the appointment, it might be worth changing that anxiety to strong concern about what the doctor may find. To do this, we will need to change that irrational demand to something like "It would be highly preferable to go to the doctor," but there is no reason saying I absolutely have to, and if I get news I don't want, it would be really bad but not terrible, and I could stand it. (Criterion 2)

Example Response to Advanced Client Statement 5

From what you're saying, it sounds like you're jealous because your boyfriend is paying more attention to his coworker than he is with you, and he seems to be enjoying her company more. I hear two beliefs that may be contributing to your jealousy. The first is an irrational belief in the form of a demand, such as "He shouldn't be spending so much time with her and he should be paying more attention to me." The other derivative irrational belief is "I'm not good enough." (Criterion 1) If you want to replace your unhealthy jealousy with healthier disappointment, we will need to replace the irrational demand and your rating yourself. The rational alternatives to your two beliefs would be something like, "I wish he would pay more attention to me, but there is no reason he must, and if he doesn't do so, that doesn't mean anything about me as a person, but maybe I don't have enough of something he prefers." (Criterion 2)

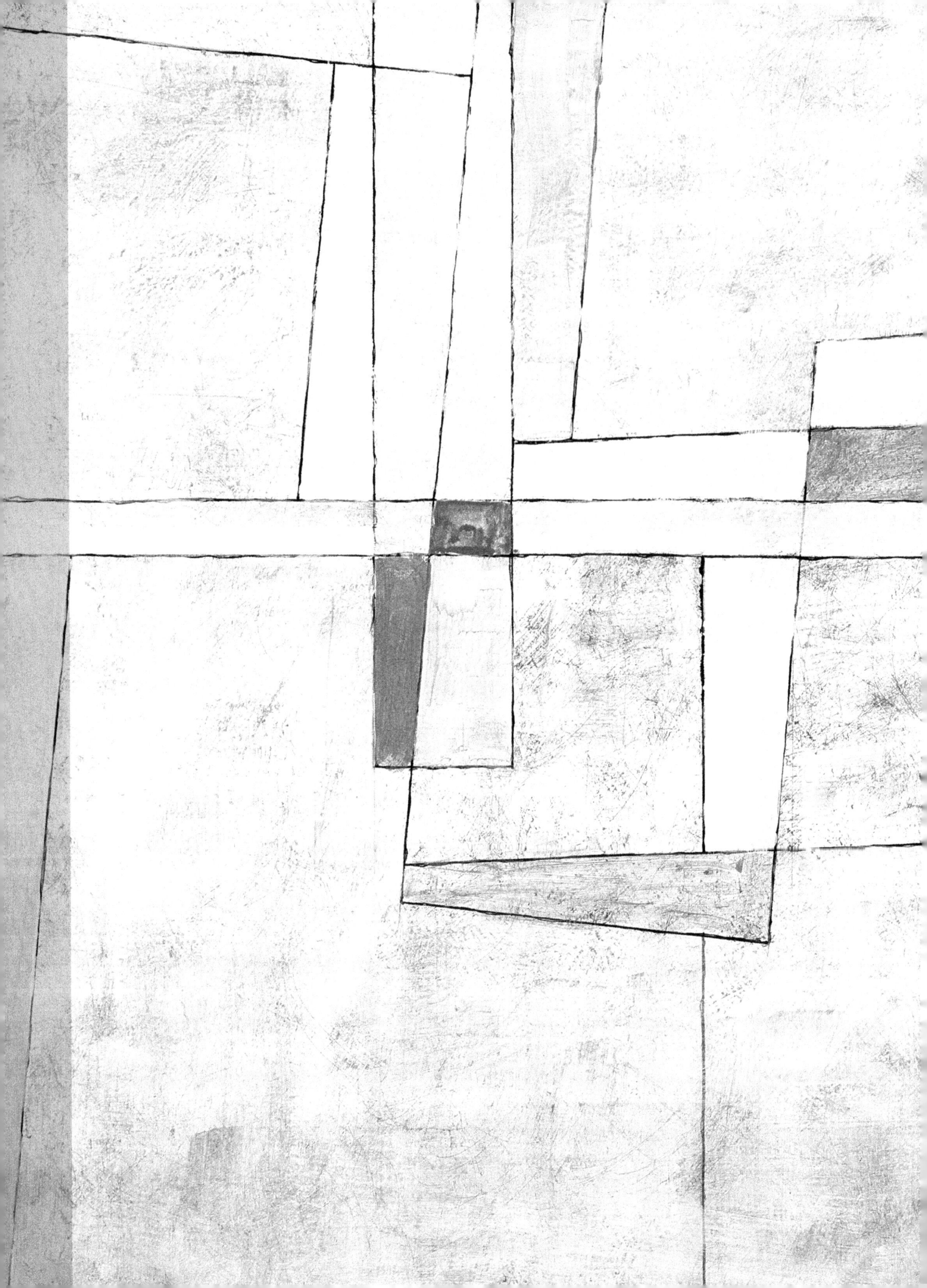

Prioritizing Which Irrational Beliefs to Target for Change

Preparations for Exercise 6

1. Read the instructions in Chapter 2.

2. Download the Deliberate Practice Reaction Form and the Deliberate Practice Diary Form at https://www.apa.org/pubs/books/deliberate-practice-rational-emotive-behavior-therapy (see the "Clinician and Practitioner Resources" tab; also available in Appendixes A and B, respectively).

Skill Description

Skill Difficulty Level: Intermediate

The goal of this exercise is to help clinicians work with clients to identify which irrational belief is contributing the most to their maladaptive or unhealthy emotional and behavioral consequences and to prioritize the sequence of irrational beliefs to target in therapy. This skill requires the clinician to consider the varied irrational beliefs that a client might hold about a specific situation (activating event) and help the client discern which one(s) create the greatest amount of disturbance (i.e., emotional or behavioral) as that will likely be the primary belief the client will want to target for change. This exercise focuses on attaining agreement on which irrational belief a client wants to work on first. The exercise assumes that the client knows and has communicated this to the therapist in their initial client statement. For rational emotive behavior therapy clinicians, we thought it important to point out that it is possible a client might not be aware of which irrational belief is most associated with their clinical problem. In such situations, the therapist would have to ask more questions concerning which irrational belief the client might endorse more strongly, which is more strongly associated with the current problem being discussed, or which one they want to work on first.

https://doi.org/10.1037/0000334-008

Deliberate Practice in Rational Emotive Behavior Therapy, by M. D. Terjesen, K. A. Doyle, R. A. DiGiuseppe, A. Vaz, and T. Rousmaniere

Special Considerations for Performing This Exercise

Please note that for the beginner difficulty level, the irrational belief(s) are presented directly in the client statements. The intermediate difficulty level will have a direct irrational belief stated and a derivative implied, or vice versa. Finally, for the advanced difficulty level, the irrational beliefs are implied but not explicitly stated. The goal is for trainees to build on the skills as clients do not always present their irrational beliefs clearly and directly.

SKILL CRITERIA FOR EXERCISE 6

1. Reflect the main irrational beliefs presented by the client.
2. Highlight the one irrational belief that appears to be the primary contributor to the unhealthy consequence.
3. Check with the client for agreement that this belief represents the primary irrational belief to be targeted for change.

Examples of Therapists Prioritizing Which Irrational Beliefs to Target for Change

Example 1

CLIENT: [*angry*] My partner constantly criticizes me and tells me to do things that she should do herself. It really infuriates me. She shouldn't say anything. She does this to me all the time! I really can't deal with this anymore. What bothers me most is that she says things she shouldn't.

THERAPIST: It sounds like there are two possible beliefs that lead you to make yourself angry when she criticizes you: "She **shouldn't** do this" and "I can't deal with this anymore!" The "should" is a demand, and the "I really can't deal with this anymore" is a frustration intolerance belief. (Criterion 1) Toward the end, you said that when she says things that she shouldn't, that is what bothers you the most. (Criterion 2) Given this, are you in agreement that, of these two beliefs, we will start with your demand of what she **shouldn't** do, that leads to your anger? (Criterion 3)

Example 2

CLIENT: [*anxious*] I am so anxious and I find myself thinking about everything that could go wrong with the charity event that it's disrupting my sleep. If it fails, that would be **terrible**. I **have to** make sure I am on top of every detail, and I can't delegate to others. But truthfully, I don't mind managing every detail as much as the idea of the event failing.

THERAPIST: Based on what you described, it sounds as if you are feeling anxious and having trouble sleeping perhaps because of the two beliefs you mentioned: One, "It would be **terrible** if this charity event went poorly," which is an awfulizing evaluation, and two "I **have to** handle every detail," which is a demandingness belief. (Criterion 1) Now, of these two beliefs, it sounds like your awfulizing belief is the one that causes you more anxiety and impacts your sleep. Is that correct? (Criterion 2) Given this, are we in agreement to begin with changing the awfulizing belief? (Criterion 3)

Example 3

CLIENT: [*depressed*] I am literally watching my mother's health deteriorate in front of me and I am so depressed and crying uncontrollably. As her daughter, I really did not do what I should have done to have gotten her the kind of care she needed earlier. I'm such a bad person and that belief really upsets me the most.

THERAPIST: When you feel depressed and have these periods of uncontrollable crying, it sounds like you have some beliefs about yourself and the situation. Might you be thinking "I should have done more to help her," which is a demand, and also globally rating yourself as a bad person? (Criterion 1) Of these two beliefs, is there one that creates more of your depression? Toward the end, you said the "bad person" belief is the one that upsets you the most. Shall we prioritize that one? (Criterion 2) OK, often, when we rate ourselves as bad people, we may experience depression. If we want to work on not having you feel depressed but instead feel a healthier negative emotion such as sadness, would you agree that it would make sense to prioritize those ratings of worth beliefs that contribute to your feelings of depression? (Criterion 3)

INSTRUCTIONS FOR EXERCISE 6

Step 1: Role-Play and Feedback

- The client says the first beginner client statement. The therapist **improvises** a response based on the skill criteria.
- The trainer (or if not available, the client) provides **brief** feedback based on the skill criteria.
- The client then repeats the same statement, and the therapist again improvises a response. The trainer (or client) again provides brief feedback.

Step 2: Repeat

- Repeat Step 1 for all the statements **in the current difficulty level** (beginner, intermediate, or advanced).

Step 3: Assess and Adjust Difficulty

- The therapist completes the Deliberate Practice Reaction Form (see Appendix A) and decides whether to make the exercise easier or harder or to repeat the same difficulty level.

Step 4: Repeat for Approximately 15 Minutes

- Repeat Steps 1 to 3 for at least 15 minutes.
- The trainees then switch therapist and client roles and start over.

Now it's your turn! Follow Steps 1 and 2 from the instructions.

Remember: The goal of the role-play is for trainees to practice improvising responses to the client statements in a manner that (a) uses the skill criteria and (b) feels authentic for the trainee. **Example therapist responses for each client statement are provided at the end of this exercise. Trainees should attempt to improvise their own responses before reading the example responses.**

BEGINNER-LEVEL CLIENT STATEMENTS FOR EXERCISE 6
Beginner Client Statement 1
[Angry] I was so angry the other day at my colleague because she never gets back to me about anything in a timely manner. I can't stand it when I see she has read my text or emails. Is it that tough to respond? She should at least tell me she will get to it soon! That is the part that upsets me the most. I vent about her to my partner daily!
Beginner Client Statement 2
[Depressed] I have always gotten positive reviews at work, but I did not this year. I should have known that with a new supervisor I had to change what I was doing. I am such an idiot. Everyone knows I screwed up, and then I stopped doing what was needed to get a better review. That "I am an idiot" statement keeps going through my head the most.
Beginner Client Statement 3
[Guilty] I told my friend that he could not stay with me because we were having other houseguests, which wasn't true. He ended up staying at some dive hotel and almost got robbed. I should have let him stay. I am such a lousy friend and a really bad person. Who does that to someone? I feel so guilty and when I feel this way, I think about being such a lousy person.
Beginner Client Statement 4
[Anxious] If I don't pass this course, I will have to go to summer school. That would be the worst thing to have to deal with. While all my friends can go to the beach or have jobs, I will be stuck in a classroom, and the idea is intolerable. I haven't even been able to study because I am so stressed and anxious. My head is full of "worst" and "can't stand it" thoughts, but there are more times when I am anxious that I am thinking this would be the worst.
Beginner Client Statement 5
[Jealous] Why does my boss keep praising him when I did all the work? I should have the attention and approval he gets. My boss probably likes him better and will now promote him. I am so envious of the attention and credit he gets. I should get the proper credit here and should get the promotion he is going to get. This happens all the time, and I'm starting to think I'm inadequate. Those "shoulds" keep going through my head all the time. I heard a rumor that he has done some unsavory things. I am going to tell my boss about this.

🛑 **Assess and adjust the difficulty before moving to the next difficulty level (see Step 3 in the exercise instructions).**

INTERMEDIATE-LEVEL CLIENT STATEMENTS FOR EXERCISE 6
Intermediate Client Statement 1
[Angry] I get that I am not perfect, but while driving back with our friends from vacation, she criticized me the whole time. I was fuming mad and was ready to break something. She shouldn't criticize me in front of others! I didn't blow up in front of the others, but I did when I got home. I told her, "Don't you ever do that again!" This is enough public criticism!
Intermediate Client Statement 2
[Depressed] I thought for sure I nailed this job interview, yet I didn't get it despite all of my experience. Obviously, there is something about me that I can't get hired. I am such a loser. I just want to give up and change careers.
Intermediate Client Statement 3
[Guilty] I feel so guilty I cannot work. I took credit for work that I really didn't do, and I know I shouldn't have. It was a group project, but I barely pulled my share of the work. There's got to be something about me to have done this. When I think about this, I get paralyzed and I can't do anything.
Intermediate Client Statement 4
[Anxious] I am debating whether I can really take this promotion. If I do it and fail, it will be a colossal disaster and be terrible. Why would I want to face this anxiety? With this anxiety, I don't even think I will try.
Intermediate Client Statement 5
[Jealous] I put more preparation into the pitch meeting than he did, and he just makes a quip, and they all fall head-over-heels for his idea. I should have the same degree of skill, which would get me the recognition that he has, but I don't, which has to say something about me. This is my dream job, but I will always be in his shadow unless I leave and go somewhere else.

 Assess and adjust the difficulty before moving to the next difficulty level (see Step 3 in the exercise instructions).

ADVANCED-LEVEL CLIENT STATEMENTS FOR EXERCISE 6

Advanced Client Statement 1

[Angry] I gave what I believe to be very clear directions, and she did not follow them. She then tried to blame me and make me look bad. I was so furious at that that I threw a book down and cracked the glass table. Treat me with some respect!

Advanced Client Statement 2

[Depressed] I try and try to manage my weight and engage in healthier behaviors, but no matter what I do, I can never seem to be fit. I give in way too easily when tempted by unhealthy foods. The idea of exercising regularly is really hard and not appealing to me. I have my cousin's wedding coming up and I am thinking of not going. What does it say about me that I can't say "no" to certain foods, don't do something like light exercise, and that I can't seem to get healthy?

Advanced Client Statement 3

[Guilty] I seem to repeatedly choose work over family, which I know is wrong. What kind of a person makes choices like this? I feel so guilty all the time, and then I either avoid my family or overcompensate and do something that isn't practical or financially feasible to try and make up for it.

Advanced Client Statement 4

[Anxious] In all honesty, I could have graduated 2 years ago. Every time I think about doing my schoolwork, I avoid it because it's really difficult and I also am anxious that I might not do it correctly and may either fail or have to make substantial rewrites, which would be really bad.

Advanced Client Statement 5

[Jealous] Everyone used to look to me to coordinate any big events. Now, they all want to hold off on decisions until she weighs in. I have done a really good job and was always given credit, but now they want to give her this "planning crown," which is rightfully mine, and this makes me wonder about myself. It gets me so upset, and I want to drop out of any future events with this group.

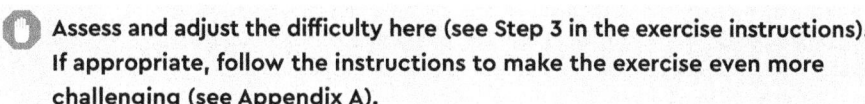 **Assess and adjust the difficulty here (see Step 3 in the exercise instructions). If appropriate, follow the instructions to make the exercise even more challenging (see Appendix A).**

Example Therapist Responses: Prioritizing Which Irrational Beliefs to Target for Change

Remember: Trainees should attempt to improvise their own responses before reading the example responses. **Do not read the following responses verbatim unless you are having trouble coming up with your own responses!**

EXAMPLE RESPONSES TO BEGINNER-LEVEL CLIENT STATEMENTS FOR EXERCISE 6
Example Response to Beginner Client Statement 1
I am hearing two possible beliefs that may lead you to make yourself so angry when she doesn't get back to you: "She shouldn't do this" and "I can't stand this!" (Criterion 1) I imagine that of the two beliefs, when you are the angriest and venting to your partner, there is one that is stronger. When you say, "She shouldn't do this," that appears to be the belief that creates the most anger for you. (Criterion 2) Does it make sense for us to work on that one first? (Criterion 3)
Example Response to Beginner Client Statement 2
It sounds as if you are depressed about your review and that you have some beliefs about your own behavior and yourself that led you to avoid doing the work: "I am such an idiot" and "I should have known or done what I needed to do to get a better review." (Criterion 1) When you are most depressed and avoid doing the work or making changes, you said that it is the "idiot" that keeps going through your head the most. (Criterion 2) By believing "I am such an idiot," you get yourself depressed the most. Should we look at changing that belief first? (Criterion 3)
Example Response to Beginner Client Statement 3
I'm wondering if you feel guilty about your decision to lie to your friend. I heard you say, "I should have let him stay" and that you are "a really bad person." (Criterion 1) While both beliefs may lead to guilt, of the two, there probably is one that is strongest when you feel guilty about lying to him. Based on what you said, it sounds like you think it is the global evaluation of your worth. (Criterion 2) From what you just said, it sounds like the "I am a really bad person" is the stronger belief and probably contributes more to your feeling guilty. What are your thoughts on prioritizing this one? (Criterion 3)
Example Response to Beginner Client Statement 4
If I am understanding you, the stress and anxiety you are experiencing about passing this class and avoiding studying comes from two beliefs: "Going to summer school would be the worst thing to deal with" and "Being stuck in a classroom would be intolerable." (Criterion 1) Of these two beliefs, it sounds like the one you think more strongly when you are most anxious and avoid studying is that going to summer school would be the worst thing that could happen. (Criterion 2) Does it make sense for us to work on that one first? (Criterion 3)
Example Response to Beginner Client Statement 5
From what you reported, it sounds like you are feeling jealous of your coworker. I am hearing two possible beliefs that might lead you to become jealous to the point that you want to spread rumors: "I should get the proper credit here and the promotion" and "I'm inadequate." (Criterion 1) When you are at your most jealous and thinking of spreading rumors, one of these beliefs may be stronger and as a result more problematic. And from what you say it sounds like it is the "shoulds." (Criterion 2) Does it make sense for us to work on that demanding belief first? (Criterion 3)

EXAMPLE RESPONSES TO INTERMEDIATE-LEVEL CLIENT STATEMENTS FOR EXERCISE 6

Example Response to Intermediate Client Statement 1

It sounds like you were furious and that two beliefs led to your anger and aggression. One was that "she should not criticize me in front of others," and the second was that her criticism is "too much" for you at this point. (Criterion 1) Since the "she shouldn't" belief led to anger and aggression and it was your first thought you recall experiencing, perhaps that "she shouldn't" was the more powerful thought. (Criterion 2) If you agree, might we challenge the "shouldn't" statement first? (Criterion 3)

Example Response to Intermediate Client Statement 2

From what you report, your depression is related to two beliefs: you are a "loser" and you "should have" gotten the job because of your experience. (Criterion 1) Because the "loser" belief led to your desire to quit and change careers, it could be the one that led to your upset the most. (Criterion 2) Could we agree to start by targeting that "loser" statement for change and help you adopt a more rational alternative idea? (Criterion 3)

Example Response to Intermediate Client Statement 3

You seem to have two irrational beliefs that are leading to your dysfunctional guilt. One is the demand that you should not have taken credit for the work. The second is that you are some type of subhuman because you did this thing you should not have done. (Criterion 1) It sounds to me that the global self-condemning belief leads to the dysfunctional behavior and might be the irrational belief causing you the most trouble. (Criterion 2) If that is the primary belief, should we work on changing that belief first so you can do your work and feel regret instead of guilt? (Criterion 3)

Example Response to Intermediate Client Statement 4

You seem to have overwhelming anxiety and a strong desire not even to give this job a try. It sounds like there are two beliefs that are causing you trouble. First, you're thinking that it would be terrible to fail. Second, you think you can't stand to face your anxiety. (Criterion 1) I propose that we work on the intolerance of the anxiety first, because if you do not face that, we are unlikely to get to discuss the other. (Criterion 2) Do you agree that we should try and change your belief that you can't stand facing the anxiety? (Criterion 3)

Example Response to Intermediate Client Statement 5

I hear two irrational beliefs in this situation that are leading up to your dysfunctional jealousy and your considering leaving your dream job. First, you have the belief that you should have the same degree of skill that he has. And second, you hold the belief that you are globally inadequate if you do not have the things you should have. (Criterion 1) It could be that the demand that you should be as skilled as he is the core belief that triggers the other one. (Criterion 2) Can I propose that we target this demand first in the session? (Criterion 3)

EXAMPLE RESPONSES TO ADVANCED-LEVEL CLIENT STATEMENTS FOR EXERCISE 6

Example Response to Advanced Client Statement 1

I have a hypothesis that you might have been telling yourself, "She should have followed my clear directions," "She shouldn't have blamed me for not doing so," and "She should show me some respect." (Criterion 1) The first one led to you becoming furious and throwing the book. While all these demanding beliefs may contribute to your anger and subsequent aggressive behavior, one could do so more. Based on your behavior, it sounds like the demand about how she should not blame you appears to create the most anger for you. (Criterion 2) If that's correct, would it be best if we start with this demand first? (Criterion 3)

Example Response to Advanced Client Statement 2

It sounds like you're feeling depressed about your lack of progress in getting fit and giving into eating unhealthy foods. I'm hearing three beliefs that may be self-defeating for you, one being a demand that you should be more disciplined with food and exercise, another being a frustration intolerance belief of "it's too hard to exercise regularly and say no to unhealthy foods," and another sounds like a self-condemnation belief when you ask, "What does it say about me that I can't say no to certain foods?" (Criterion 1) Of these three beliefs, one may contribute most to you feeling depressed and contemplating not going to your cousin's wedding. I could be wrong, but it sounds like your self-condemning belief is the strongest one that is contributing to your depression, and perhaps you then continue giving in to eating unhealthy foods. (Criterion 2) If this is accurate, should we start with the self-condemning belief first? (Criterion 3)

Example Response to Advanced Client Statement 3

I hear three beliefs that might be contributing to your guilt and then avoidance or overcompensation behavior. The first is a demandingness belief such as "I shouldn't choose work over family," the second is a self-downing belief such as "I'm a bad person because I do so," and the third is a frustration intolerance belief when you avoid or overcompensate because you may be thinking something like "It's too uncomfortable to deal with the consequences of my decisions." (Criterion 1) While all play a role, one of these three beliefs may be a stronger contributor to your guilt and self-defeating behaviors. Guilt may come from some self-condemnation. (Criterion 2) It sounds like we could start with the self-downing belief of being a bad person because of your choices, do you agree? (Criterion 3)

Example Response to Advanced Client Statement 4

Although you say you could have graduated 2 years ago, I'm hypothesizing that it's really a demanding belief that you should have graduated. I also hear a frustration intolerance belief that doing schoolwork is not just really difficult, but it's too difficult. Then there sounds like an awfulizing belief about doing it incorrectly and possibly failing or having to do rewrites. (Criterion 1) While all these beliefs probably result in anxiety and avoidance behaviors, one may be contributing more. It sounds like if you didn't awfulize about the potential outcome you would be more likely to get down to doing the work because you wouldn't feel anxiety. (Criterion 2) Is working on changing this awfulizing belief where we should start? (Criterion 3)

Example Response to Advanced Client Statement 5

I'm wondering if you're thinking you should be getting the credit rather than her, and because you're not, somehow that makes you not good enough as a person. I also wonder if you have a frustration intolerance belief such as it's too unbearable to see her get the credit. (Criterion 1) These beliefs all may result in a feeling of jealousy toward this woman and wanting to drop out of future events with one belief possibly being stronger than the other two. (Criterion 2) Often, jealousy can begin with a demandingness belief of what we think we should be getting. If you do have a "should" belief about getting credit and that is what leads to you feeling jealous, would that be where you think we would be best served to start? (Criterion 3)

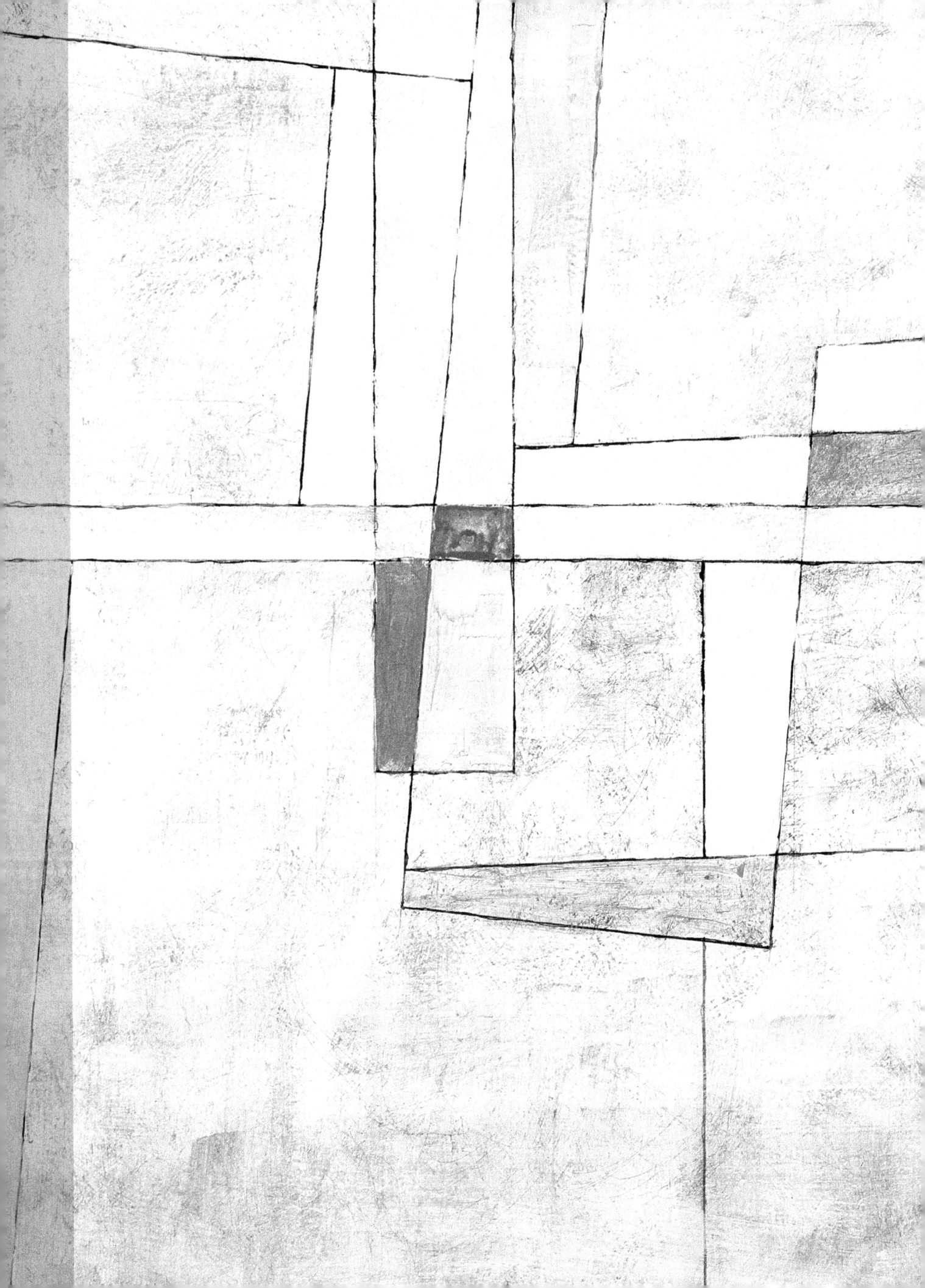

Teaching the Belief–Consequence Connection

Preparations for Exercise 7

1. Read the instructions in Chapter 2.

2. Download the Deliberate Practice Reaction Form and the Deliberate Practice Diary Form at https://www.apa.org/pubs/books/deliberate-practice-rational-emotive-behavior-therapy (see the "Clinician and Practitioner Resources" tab; also available in Appendixes A and B, respectively).

Skill Description

Skill Difficulty Level: Intermediate

Rational emotive behavior therapy (REBT) proposes that clients' beliefs (the Bs from the ABC model described in Exercise 1) are important in determining their emotional and behavioral problems or consequences (Cs). This theory dates back in part to the Stoic philosophers, such as Epictetus, who famously stated, "People are disturbed not by things but by their view of things." While there are some similarities between Stoic philosophy and REBT, there are also some important differences (DiGiuseppe et al., 2014). A contemporary REBT adaptation of Epictetus's dictum could be: "People disturb themselves by the rigid and extreme beliefs that they hold about things" (Dryden, David, & Ellis, 2010, p. 226).

The goal of this exercise is to help clinicians teach clients the belief and consequence (B–C) connection. This skill is among the more important ones within the REBT framework, as it teaches clients the connection between their irrational belief and their unhealthy consequences (Cs, which include negative disturbed, affective/emotional states and their maladaptive behaviors). Understanding that the beliefs that a client experiences lead to these consequences is essential before the therapist disputes (challenges) these beliefs.

https://doi.org/10.1037/0000334-009

Deliberate Practice in Rational Emotive Behavior Therapy, by M. D. Terjesen, K. A. Doyle, R. A. DiGiuseppe, A. Vaz, and T. Rousmaniere

SKILL CRITERIA FOR EXERCISE 7
1. Make a statement that connects the client's irrational belief with its consequence (C).
2. Ask a question that checks the client's understanding of the B–C connection.

Examples of Therapists Teaching the Belief–Consequence Connection

Example 1

CLIENT: [*angry*] My boss makes me so pissed off when she repeatedly forgets that she told me something and then checks my progress after I have already told her this. She does it all the time, and I really can't deal with it. A boss should do her job!

THERAPIST: It sounds like you are getting yourself angry when you think, "I can't deal with her behavior, and she should do her job!" Is that correct? (Criterion 1) Do you understand that as long as you think "and I can't stand this," you are going to continue to make yourself angry? (Criterion 2)

Example 2

CLIENT: [*anxious*] I am so worried about the third round of interviews for this job. I am happy I made it this far, but now I am stressed because I really want this job, and if I screw up the interview, that would be pretty terrible. I struggle with sleep because I keep thinking about how I might not make it this far again in the interview process, and if I don't get this job, I might have to move back with my parents or go on unemployment, which would be awful.

THERAPIST: It sounds like you have difficulty sleeping because you are causing yourself to get anxious by thinking about how awful and terrible it would be if you don't get this job. Is that correct? (Criterion 1) Do you see the connection between your "awful" and "terrible" beliefs and your feelings of anxiety and difficulty sleeping? (Criterion 2)

Example 3

CLIENT: [*depressed*] This is now the third relationship I've had in the last year that ended with the person breaking up with me. It's clearly about me. What's wrong with me? I don't think anyone will ever want to be with me because I am such an idiot and a loser. This makes me so upset that I just want to curl into a ball and cry. I was so depressed that I canceled plans with friends and called out sick for work for 2 days.

THERAPIST: It sounds like when you feel depressed, you are engaging in a lot of ratings about yourself, thinking "I am no good, am an idiot, a loser" and "No one will care about me because I am worthless." These thoughts also then lead to you avoiding important things, like social outings and work. Is that correct? (Criterion 1) Do you see the connection between your thinking "I'm such an idiot and a loser" and your feeling depressed and avoidance of social and work-related activities? (Criteria 2)

INSTRUCTIONS FOR EXERCISE 7

Step 1: Role-Play and Feedback

- The client says the first beginner client statement. The therapist **improvises** a response based on the skill criteria.
- The trainer (or if not available, the client) provides **brief** feedback based on the skill criteria.
- The client then repeats the same statement, and the therapist again improvises a response. The trainer (or client) again provides brief feedback.

Step 2: Repeat

- Repeat Step 1 for all the statements **in the current difficulty level** (beginner, intermediate, or advanced).

Step 3: Assess and Adjust Difficulty

- The therapist completes the Deliberate Practice Reaction Form (see Appendix A) and decides whether to make the exercise easier or harder or to repeat the same difficulty level.

Step 4: Repeat for Approximately 15 Minutes

- Repeat Steps 1 to 3 for at least 15 minutes.
- The trainees then switch therapist and client roles and start over.

> **Now it's your turn! Follow Steps 1 and 2 from the instructions.**

Remember: The goal of the role-play is for trainees to practice improvising responses to the client statements in a manner that (a) uses the skill criteria and (b) feels authentic for the trainee. **Example therapist responses for each client statement are provided at the end of this exercise. Trainees should attempt to improvise their own responses before reading the example responses.**

BEGINNER-LEVEL CLIENT STATEMENTS FOR EXERCISE 7
Beginner Client Statement 1
[Angry] I was so angry the other day because my brother had me go to pick him up at the airport, then never told me he took another flight. Now I'm not talking to him. I can't stand that he does this.
Beginner Client Statement 2
[Depressed] I really had thought we were closer friends and was very depressed that I wasn't invited to her wedding. I'm a loser and so stupid for thinking anyone would care about me like this. I don't even reach out to anyone from our friend group now.
Beginner Client Statement 3
[Guilty] I forgot to call my mother on her birthday and feel so guilty. Who knows how many more she will have? I should have called. I am such a bad person, and now I just ordered an expensive "make-up" gift that I can't afford.
Beginner Client Statement 4
[Anxious] This presentation could make or break our business. If it doesn't go well, it would be the worst thing to have to deal with, and I get so anxious when I think about it. I haven't slept well in the last 2 nights.
Beginner Client Statement 5
[Jealous] Why is my boyfriend giving her so much attention? He probably likes her and is afraid to tell me. He should be paying attention to me; I'm his girlfriend! Now I'm going to keep checking his phone.

 Assess and adjust the difficulty before moving to the next difficulty level (see Step 3 in the exercise instructions).

INTERMEDIATE-LEVEL CLIENT STATEMENTS FOR EXERCISE 7

Intermediate Client Statement 1

[Angry] I had asked if they were coming to the charity fundraiser and they said "yes." I fully expected them to be there, and they didn't show up and didn't even bother to call. I would have called. I am so livid right now and won't even talk to them!

Intermediate Client Statement 2

[Depressed] Every time I think I did well on the test, it turns out I did poorly. I am obviously not smart and not a good judge of my abilities. I don't even want to bother trying anymore. I mean, why should I? I am pretty much not good at anything!

Intermediate Client Statement 3

[Guilty] Clearly, I let her down and hurt her. I've done such a terrible thing. It was my fault and I feel so bad I can't even face her, and I'm ignoring all her efforts to connect with me.

Intermediate Client Statement 4

[Anxious] If I ask her out on a date and she says no, everyone will know, and that would be really, really bad. Just the idea of rejection is tough but having everyone know about it would be too much to handle, so I won't even ask her.

Intermediate Client Statement 5

[Jealous] No matter how hard I try, I am never going to be as good of an athlete as they are, and they will always get more attention and support from the coaches than I do. I do all the right things in practice, and they put no effort in. I'm never going to be good enough. I'm thinking of quitting the team.

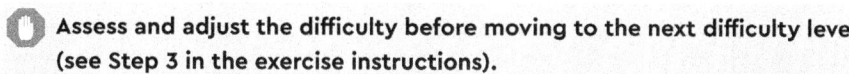 **Assess and adjust the difficulty before moving to the next difficulty level (see Step 3 in the exercise instructions).**

ADVANCED-LEVEL CLIENT STATEMENTS FOR EXERCISE 7
Advanced Client Statement 1
[Angry] It's one thing when someone doesn't do something that they say they are going to do, but it is quite another when they lie about it to your face and to other people to make you look bad. I would never do that. I don't condone fighting, but I am so angry right now at what they did, I may want to punch them.
Advanced Client Statement 2
[Depressed] I see all their posts on social media, and they clearly planned this event without me, and it seems like they are having such fun. I know I can be difficult sometimes, but I didn't realize that they really thought so little of me. Maybe they are right. I'm going to unfriend them all.
Advanced Client Statement 3
[Guilty] I am not sure what to do. Making a mistake is one thing, but this was a huge one. I feel so bad about what I did, and I am not sure I can face myself and look in the mirror. I can't even look her in the eyes.
Advanced Client Statement 4
[Anxious] This will be the second time I have had to retake this exam, and you only get two chances. What if I fail? I will be out of the training program, and this will mean I have wasted all these years and money. I cannot think of a worse thing that could happen to me. I keep postponing preparing for the exam because failing would be too much to deal with.
Advanced Client Statement 5
[Jealous] I was raised in a home where you were told to keep your personal accomplishments to yourself. So when I see her flaunting all that she's done, I think she may get promoted into my job. I get really upset and want to do something mean to her.

 Assess and adjust the difficulty here (see Step 3 in the exercise instructions). If appropriate, follow the instructions to make the exercise even more challenging (see Appendix A).

Example Therapist Responses: Teaching the Belief–Consequence Connection

Remember: Trainees should attempt to improvise their own responses before reading the example responses. **Do not read the following responses verbatim unless you are having trouble coming up with your own responses!**

EXAMPLE RESPONSES TO BEGINNER-LEVEL
CLIENT STATEMENTS FOR EXERCISE 7

Example Response to Beginner Client Statement 1

It sounds like when you think, "I can't stand that he does this," it leads you to get so angry, and now you are not even speaking to your brother. Is that correct? (Criterion 1) Does that connection of your thoughts to your feelings of anger make sense to you? (Criterion 2)

Example Response to Beginner Client Statement 2

As we have discussed, in REBT we want to look at how our unhealthy or irrational beliefs create unhealthy emotions and behaviors. Correct me if I am wrong, but it sounds like you are thinking "I'm a loser," and that makes you feel very depressed and disconnected from your friend group. Is that right? (Criterion 1) Do you understand how thinking that way will lead to those unhealthy negative emotions and behaviors? (Criterion 2)

Example Response to Beginner Client Statement 3

Unhealthy negative emotions and behaviors come from unhealthy or irrational beliefs. In what you described, it sounds like when you think "I should have called," you end up feeling so guilty and now have put yourself in a position where you are ordering gifts that you cannot afford. Is that correct? (Criterion 1) In thinking about this, do you recognize how thinking "I should have called" will lead to you feeling guilty (an unhealthy negative emotion), and then you end up doing unhealthy behaviors like buying expensive gifts that you can't really afford? (Criterion 2)

Example Response to Beginner Client Statement 4

From what you have told me, I hear that you are anxious and, as a result, you also are having difficulties sleeping? It sounds like when you think "This would be the worst thing to have to deal with," that thought leads you to experience anxiety and have sleep troubles. Am I understanding that connection correctly? (Criterion 1) Does that connection of your "worst thing" thoughts leading to your feelings of anxiety and compromised sleep make sense to you? (Criterion 2)

Example Response to Beginner Client Statement 5

The emotion of jealousy you describe and the behavior of checking his phone are probably driven by the thought "He should be paying attention to me!" Do those pieces fit together correctly for you? (Criterion 1) In thinking about these feelings and behaviors, do you understand how thinking "He should be paying attention to me!" will lead to you feeling jealous (an unhealthy negative emotion), and then you end up doing unhealthy behaviors like checking his phone, which may harm the relationship? (Criterion 2)

EXAMPLE RESPONSES TO INTERMEDIATE-LEVEL CLIENT STATEMENTS FOR EXERCISE 7

Example Response to Intermediate Client Statement 1

It sounds like you are very angry and are avoiding your friends. Yes, it was rude and inconsiderate of them not to call you and tell you that they were not coming. Could it be that you are having the thought that "they should have done the right thing and called me"? And that thought resulted in your anger? (Criterion 1) Do you see how that demand that they do the right thing would have resulted in your being so angry? (Criterion 2)

Example Response to Intermediate Client Statement 2

You sound depressed about your doing poorly on these tests and say you want to give up. Perhaps you might be thinking, "Because I'm doing poorly, I am a loser." (Criterion 1) Does it make sense to you that this type of belief could have made you depressed about doing poorly? (Criteria 2)

Example Response to Intermediate Client Statement 3

It sounds like you are feeling guilty and ignoring her even though she has reached out to you. This could be because you are condemning yourself as a total loser for your mistake. (Criterion 1) Does the idea that you are having self-condemnation beliefs that lead to your guilt make sense to you? (Criterion 2)

Example Response to Intermediate Client Statement 4

It sounds like you have anxiety about asking her out and are worried about what other people will think of you if you are rejected. Might your anxiety stem from the belief that you cannot stand everyone else knowing you were rejected? (Criterion 1) What do you think about the idea that it's the belief you could not stand other people knowing that makes you anxious? (Criterion 2)

Example Response to Intermediate Client Statement 5

You sound very despondent and depressed about how you're doing, and these emotions are leading to your quitting. Could it be that the belief your athletic skills are linked to your self-worth leads you to condemn yourself for not being as good as the others? (Criterion 1) Do you agree that such evaluation of your worth based on your athletic skill can lead to your depression? (Criterion 2)

EXAMPLE RESPONSES TO ADVANCED-LEVEL CLIENT STATEMENTS FOR EXERCISE 7

Example Response to Advanced Client Statement 1

What it sounds like I am hearing is that you are getting yourself very angry to the point where you even are considering getting aggressive. Is there a belief behind that, such as "They shouldn't behave that way"? (Criterion 1) Although what they may have done is wrong, do you see how thinking that they shouldn't act that way causes you to feel angry and consider aggression? (Criterion 2)

Example Response to Advanced Client Statement 2

When you say "Maybe they are right," that sounds like you are beating yourself up and putting yourself down, and those beliefs of "I'm not good enough" lead you to feeling depressed and start unfriending them. (Criterion 1) Do you understand how those beliefs can cause feelings of depression and also lead to unhealthy behaviors? (Criterion 2)

Example Response to Advanced Client Statement 3

While you may have made a mistake, and this may even be a big one, it sounds like you have some beliefs like "I should not have made this mistake" and "I am such an idiot for having made this mistake" that lead to you feeling guilty and avoiding her. Is that accurate? (Criterion 1) Does the idea that these self-condemnation beliefs lead to these guilty feelings and behaviors make sense to you? (Criterion 2)

Example Response to Advanced Client Statement 4

While you did not say this, it sounds like you are experiencing a good deal of anxiety. This anxiety, and your avoidant behavior of postponing preparing, stems from some unhealthy or irrational beliefs, such as "This would be terrible to have to deal with." Am I understanding that connection correctly? (Criterion 1) Does that connection of these "worst thing" beliefs leading to your feelings of anxiety and postponing preparation make sense to you? (Criterion 2)

Example Response to Advanced Client Statement 5

You describe being upset, but I hear more of an emotion of jealousy. Do you think the jealousy and your desire to do something mean to her is driven by the belief "She shouldn't be doing this and shouldn't get the promotion"? (Criterion 1) Does it make sense that when you are thinking "she shouldn't flaunt her accomplishments and get the promotion," this will lead you to feeling jealous (an unhealthy negative emotion), and then you end up potentially doing unhealthy behaviors like doing something mean to her? (Criterion 2)

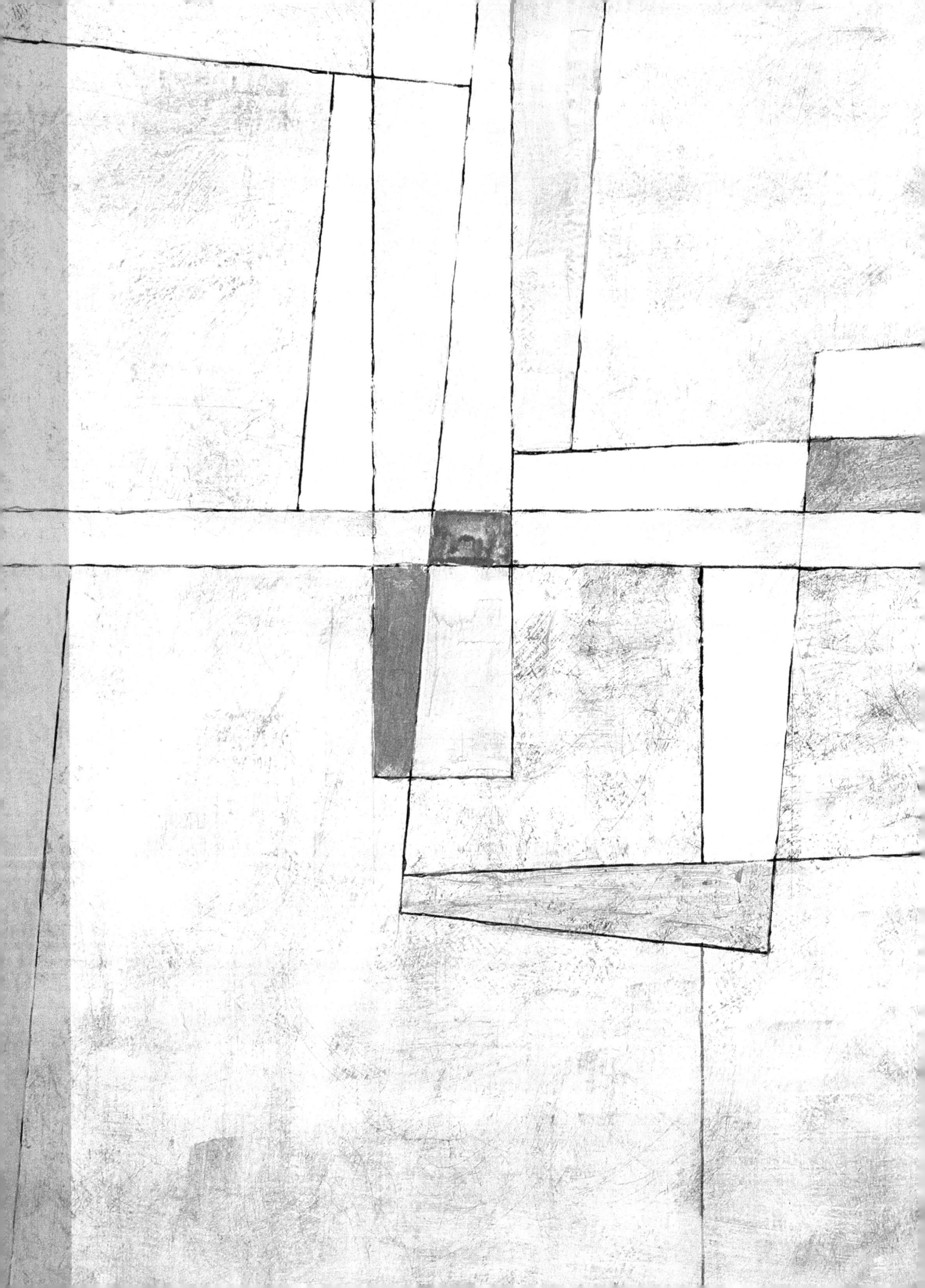

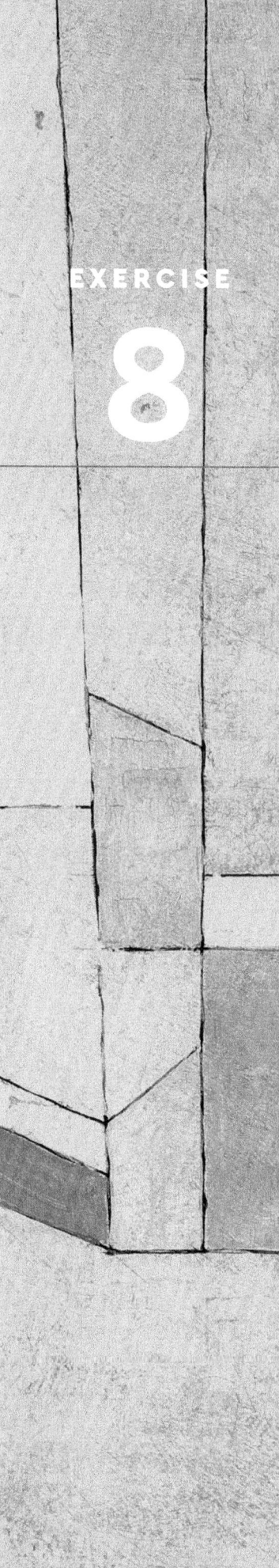

Functional Disputation of Irrational Beliefs

Preparations for Exercise 8

1. Read the instructions in Chapter 2.

2. Download the Deliberate Practice Reaction Form and the Deliberate Practice Diary Form at https://www.apa.org/pubs/books/deliberate-practice-rational-emotive-behavior-therapy (see the "Clinician and Practitioner Resources" tab; also available in Appendixes A and B, respectively).

Skill Description

Skill Difficulty Level: Intermediate

Disputing, questioning, or challenging clients' irrational beliefs is an activity that rational emotive behavior therapy (REBT) posits will produce a change in the client. An effective REBT clinician will become proficient in the application of multiple disputation strategies. This exercise and the next two focus on a different disputation strategy but will be using the same client prompts. One of the core disputation strategies is referred to as a *functional* or *pragmatic disputation*. In this, the REBT clinician works with the client to determine whether their irrational belief(s) are helping them to achieve their stated goal(s). In so doing, the clinician challenges the clients' irrational beliefs that lead to maladaptive/unhealthy emotions and dysfunctional behaviors. The skill in this exercise requires the clinician to (a) consider the irrational belief(s) that the client holds about a specific situation, (b) summarize with the client what that belief is, (c) ask questions about whether holding the belief results in the client achieving their goals or blocks the client from achieving their goals, and (d) check with the client for understanding of how that belief works against their clinical goals.

Very often irrational beliefs may be implied when the client asks an open-ended question. For example, "What kind of person am I to have done something like that to

https://doi.org/10.1037/0000334-010

Deliberate Practice in Rational Emotive Behavior Therapy, by M. D. Terjesen, K. A. Doyle, R. A. DiGiuseppe, A. Vaz, and T. Rousmaniere

her?" This question implies that because they behaved a certain way, the client may think poorly of themselves, and we would categorize this as ratings of worth. A skilled REBT clinician will listen for the implied irrational belief behind a question and propose it as an irrational belief of the client that may be contributing to their emotional and behavioral difficulties. In the advanced client statements, we have added a number of comments like this to promote trainees' ability to identify an irrational belief of an implied comment or question.

Special Considerations for Performing This Exercise

In this exercise, we differentiate the three skill levels (beginner, intermediate, and advanced) in the following manner: For the beginner prompts, clients directly provide one irrational belief; for the intermediate prompts, clients explicitly provide two irrational beliefs; and for the advanced prompts, clients explicitly provide one irrational belief and a second irrational belief that is implied for the clinician to propose what the belief is. We also make this differentiation in skills for the three examples after the skill criteria.

SKILL CRITERIA FOR EXERCISE 8
1. Highlight the main irrational beliefs presented by the client.
2. Challenge the client's irrational beliefs using a functional approach.
3. Check that the client understands that their irrational beliefs are working against their clinical goals.

Examples of Therapists Using Functional Disputation of Irrational Beliefs

Example 1

CLIENT: [*angry*] My mother offers her contrary opinion all the time. She shouldn't do this. I would not do this to her, and I end up yelling at her. Really, I don't like feeling this way toward her; I'd prefer to feel really annoyed with her but get along with her better.

THERAPIST: You say that you "don't like feeling this way toward her" and that you want to replace the anger with annoyance. In looking at the beliefs that lead to your anger, it sounds like you are thinking that because you do not like your mother's behavior, she "should not do this!" (Criterion 1) Does this demanding belief that she **should** act a certain way help you work toward your goal of feeling really annoyed toward her and avoid yelling at her? (Criterion 2) Do you see how holding this "should" belief leads you to feel anger and move away from your goal of annoyance? (Criterion 3)

Example 2

CLIENT: [*anxious*] I am quite sure my boyfriend is going to break up with me. I'm so anxious about this and clingy now, and I can't stand this feeling. I really want to feel concerned instead of anxious. If he did break up with me, it would be terrible!

THERAPIST: It sounds like your belief that "this would be terrible" is what leads to you feeling anxious and becoming very clingy. (Criterion 1) It also sounds like you do not think you can stand or tolerate this feeling of anxiety. These awfulizing beliefs as well as discomfort avoidance won't help you work toward your goal of feeling concerned instead of anxious and less clingy. (Criterion 2) If this belief about how "terrible" this would be is what causes that feeling of anxiety and clingy behavior, do you see how they are not consistent with your goals? (Criterion 3)

Example 3

CLIENT: [*depressed*] I get asked to go to the gym by my friends all the time and when I have gone, I see they all are in much better shape than I am. No matter how hard I try, I struggle to get more fit. I look at them and then I think I should be able to get in shape. I see myself not just as someone who struggles at the gym, but I also ask myself what's wrong with me and so I've stopped going. Going only makes me feel more depressed. I wish I could go to the gym and be with my friends, and when I see them, I'd rather be sad that it is more of a struggle for me, but not depressed.

THERAPIST: I hear some demandingness with the belief "I should be able to get into shape" but also a lot of self-condemnation with the belief "I see myself as a failure as a person." (Criterion 1) I imagine that demandingness doesn't help you get in shape at all and that those self-condemnation beliefs do not help you work toward your goal of feeling sadness and increase your going to the gym with others? (Criterion 2) Do you understand that those "should" statements and self-condemnation beliefs make your goals more difficult to attain? (Criterion 3)

INSTRUCTIONS FOR EXERCISE 8

Step 1: Role-Play and Feedback

- The client says the first beginner client statement. The therapist **improvises** a response based on the skill criteria.
- The trainer (or if not available, the client) provides **brief** feedback based on the skill criteria.
- The client then repeats the same statement, and the therapist again improvises a response. The trainer (or client) again provides brief feedback.

Step 2: Repeat

- Repeat Step 1 for all the statements **in the current difficulty level** (beginner, intermediate, or advanced).

Step 3: Assess and Adjust Difficulty

- The therapist completes the Deliberate Practice Reaction Form (see Appendix A) and decides whether to make the exercise easier or harder or to repeat the same difficulty level.

Step 4: Repeat for Approximately 15 Minutes

- Repeat Steps 1 to 3 for at least 15 minutes.
- The trainees then switch therapist and client roles and start over.

Now it's your turn! Follow Steps 1 and 2 from the instructions.

Remember: The goal of the role-play is for trainees to practice improvising responses to the client statements in a manner that (a) uses the skill criteria and (b) feels authentic for the trainee. **Example therapist responses for each client statement are provided at the end of this exercise. Trainees should attempt to improvise their own responses before reading the example responses.**

BEGINNER-LEVEL CLIENT STATEMENTS FOR EXERCISE 8
Beginner Client Statement 1
[Angry] My anger was through the roof, and I freaked out on her when, at the last minute, my boss dropped a bunch of work for me to do that isn't part of my job. She shouldn't assume I'm going to do it because she can't get her other staff to do their jobs. This is so unfair.
Beginner Client Statement 2
[Depressed] I continue to feel depressed when I think about my 30-year, loveless relationship. I want to get out, but this is probably the best I'll ever get because, really, I'm inadequate and see myself as worthless. I guess I'm going to stay stuck in this because in the game of life, I am a failure.
Beginner Client Statement 3
[Guilty] Technically, I have not cheated on my partner, but I have formed an emotional connection with someone else. When asked about it, I lie and say it is nothing, but I feel so guilty. I shouldn't be doing this.
Beginner Client Statement 4
[Anxious] I have to go to a wedding without my long-time partner and am so anxious about people coming up to me and asking why I'm there alone. Having to answer that question would be terrible. Even though it's my close friend's wedding and I want to be there, I am thinking about not going.
Beginner Client Statement 5
[Jealous] My girlfriend seems to prefer this other guy's company over mine. I have been nothing but a good, supportive boyfriend, but now it looks like I am an afterthought. I am so jealous. No one should treat someone like that. I want to stay in this relationship, but I want to lose the jealousy.

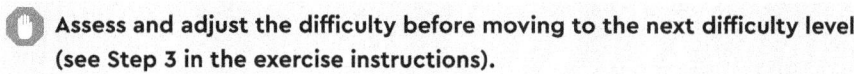 **Assess and adjust the difficulty before moving to the next difficulty level (see Step 3 in the exercise instructions).**

INTERMEDIATE-LEVEL CLIENT STATEMENTS FOR EXERCISE 8

Intermediate Client Statement 1

[Angry] We had all put in an equal amount of money for the investment property initially, but I worked on fixing the place up and put in my own money and time. Now that we're selling it, they don't want to reimburse me for this. We had a cursing argument that was so heated, it got physical and someone was thrown to the ground. They should reimburse me for the sale, and I can't stand that they're not.

Intermediate Client Statement 2

[Depressed] I exercise, I diet, but no matter what I do, I can't lose weight. I've started questioning why I'm even bothering. You would think with all this effort, it would be just as easy for me to lose weight as others, but it's not. I should be able to accomplish this goal like others can, and if I can't, that would be awful!

Intermediate Client Statement 3

[Guilty] Almost daily, I plant seeds in my colleague and friend's mind that she shouldn't apply for that promotion because I secretly want it. I know I'm acting in my own interests and that I shouldn't be sneaky and try to block her from her goals. I think I'm a horrible person for doing what I'm doing.

Intermediate Client Statement 4

[Anxious] I have this one chance to show my supervisor that I can do this project. However, I am so anxious about failing that I've been avoiding getting started. I want to prove myself and if I don't and I fail at it, it would be awful and the worst thing that has ever happened to me. If I fail, it would also prove I'm totally incompetent.

Intermediate Client Statement 5

[Jealous] Why do my parents see my brother as the golden child and always favor him over me? I should get to be in the spotlight sometimes and get some recognition for my accomplishments. I can't stand that they always overlook me.

 Assess and adjust the difficulty before moving to the next difficulty level (see Step 3 in the exercise instructions).

ADVANCED-LEVEL CLIENT STATEMENTS FOR EXERCISE 8

Advanced Client Statement 1

[Angry] I was told that the promotion was mine. They then went and hired someone with far less experience than I have, and no one could give me a reason. I was so furious that I lost it and began yelling at them in front of other staffers. They should stick to their word! What kind of people do these things?!

Advanced Client Statement 2

[Depressed] I am so depressed. I noticed that once I retired, all the people who I thought were my friends were just coworkers. No one showed up at my birthday happy hour, which confirms I'm a loser. Why don't I have more of a personality so that others would want to hang out with me?

Advanced Client Statement 3

[Guilty] I am left thinking I should have done more for my mother during her final few months, but I didn't. Every time I think about what I did—or actually, what I didn't do— I feel so guilty. What does that say about me that I didn't do that? I try not to think about her because I feel so guilty.

Advanced Client Statement 4

[Anxious] We haven't spent time together in years, and what if it's awkward? What if I have nothing to say? That would be awful and unbearable. This scenario is not something I'm up for. I'm most likely going to cancel.

Advanced Client Statement 5

[Jealous] Every big professional opportunity seems to go to this one coworker. My reviews are good, so I should be offered some of these opportunities too. Maybe I'm incompetent and that's why I keep getting passed over. We used to be close, but now it's every woman for herself!

 Assess and adjust the difficulty here (see Step 3 in the exercise instructions). If appropriate, follow the instructions to make the exercise even more challenging (see Appendix A).

Example Therapist Responses: Functional Disputation of Irrational Beliefs

Remember: Trainees should attempt to improvise their own responses before reading the example responses. **Do not read the following responses verbatim unless you are having trouble coming up with your own responses!**

EXAMPLE RESPONSES TO BEGINNER-LEVEL CLIENT STATEMENTS FOR EXERCISE 8
Example Response to Beginner Client Statement 1
When we discussed goals, we agreed on working on changing your anger to strong annoyance. We pinpointed that the belief she "shouldn't do this" is what leads to your anger. (Criterion 1) How does this demanding belief help you work towards your goal of feeling strong annoyance rather than anger? (Criterion 2) If anything, can you see how this "should" is actually creating your anger and hurting your ability to achieve your goal? (Criterion 3)
Example Response to Beginner Client Statement 2
As your goal is to break out of this cycle of depression, let's examine the belief that "I'm inadequate, worthless, and a failure" that leads to your depression. (Criterion 1) How do these global negative ratings of yourself help you work toward your goal of feeling sad about your current relationship? (Criterion 2) Do you understand that those beliefs make your goal of getting unstuck more difficult to attain? (Criterion 3)
Example Response to Beginner Client Statement 3
You stated that your goal was to replace feeling guilty about your behavior with healthier remorse. It sounds like the belief that "I shouldn't be doing this to him" makes you feel guilty. (Criterion 1) How does this demanding belief about what you have been doing help you work toward your goal of feeling regret instead of guilt? (Criterion 2) Can you understand how this demanding belief actually makes it more difficult for you to achieve your goal? (Criterion 3)
Example Response to Beginner Client Statement 4
To address your anxiety, let's examine the belief that "it would be horrible if I had to tell people why I was alone at the wedding." (Criterion 1) Given your stated goal of attending the wedding and feeling concerned instead of anxious, how does the belief of thinking it would be horrible to explain why you're alone help you work toward your goal? (Criterion 2) If anything, do you understand that this awfulizing belief hurts your movement toward that goal? (Criterion 3)
Example Response to Beginner Client Statement 5
If you want to work on giving up the jealousy, let's examine and challenge these beliefs of how she should treat you and that you are not good enough. (Criterion 1) With your goal of feeling sadness about her behavior toward you rather than jealousy, how does this demanding belief about her behavior help you work toward your goal? Does questioning your adequacy as a person help you have a good relationship with your girlfriend? (Criterion 2) If anything, can you see how these beliefs are actually creating jealousy and may harm your ability to move toward that goal of maintaining your relationship? (Criterion 3)

EXAMPLE RESPONSES TO INTERMEDIATE-LEVEL CLIENT STATEMENTS FOR EXERCISE 8

Example Response to Intermediate Client Statement 1

It sounds like you're really angry about your "partners" having stiffed you on the money you spent for upgrades to the property. We agreed that you wanted to change your anger to a healthier negative emotion of strong annoyance, which could help you pursue your grievance assertively with your partners. You identified that it is the belief that you can't stand that they did this as well as the demand that they must not behave unfairly that's creating your anger. (Criterion 1) Does demanding your partners be fair when they're not and thinking that you cannot stand it help you to be assertive with them? (Criterion 2) Does believing that you can't stand it help you have strong annoyance and maintain your resolve and perseverance? Do you think holding on to the idea that you can't stand it and that they "must" do the right thing will help you be persuasive in getting them to reimburse you? (Criterion 3)

Example Response to Intermediate Client Statement 2

You have the demand that you should be able to lose weight and the belief that if you cannot, that would be awful, which is probably what is creating your depression. (Criterion 1) How does continuing to tell yourself that you should be able to lose weight help you to feel better and do your best to lose weight? Can you see how believing it would be awful if you don't lose weight only gets in the way of your goal? (Criterion 2) I am not sure that you can lose the weight you want, but can you tell me how having that demand, and believing it would be awful if you can't lose weight, will help you get to the weight you want to be? (Criterion 3)

Example Response to Intermediate Client Statement 3

It sounds like the belief that you shouldn't be acting this way and that you are a horrible person is what is causing your guilt. (Criterion 1) Can you see how holding on to the belief that you shouldn't be acting this way toward your colleague and you're a horrible person for doing so is hurting you? (Criterion 2) Do you understand that this demand and self-condemning belief is leading you to feel guilty and not work toward your goal? (Criterion 3)

Example Response to Intermediate Client Statement 4

The beliefs that failing would be awful and the worst thing that happened to you as well as "prove" that you are incompetent are probably what is resulting in your anxiety. (Criterion 1) Does telling yourself that if you fail it would be awful and the end of the world and that would confirm that you are totally incompetent help you achieve your goals or get in the way? (Criterion 2) Can you see that if you continue to hold the beliefs that if you fail at this project, it would be the worst thing that ever happened to you and would mean you are incompetent is what contributes to you avoiding starting the project, which may in fact increase the chances that you will fail? (Criterion 3)

Example Response to Intermediate Client Statement 5

The belief about you not being able to stand their behavior as well as the demand about how they should treat you in comparison to your brother sound like they are what leads to your jealousy. (Criterion 1) Does demanding that you be in the spotlight sometimes, and you're not, help you in any way? Does thinking that you cannot stand it benefit you or change your parents' or your brother's behavior? (Criterion 2) Do you understand that this demanding belief as well as thinking that you cannot stand their behavior has not helped you have a good relationship with your parents or with your brother and perhaps has gotten in the way of you occasionally being in the spotlight? (Criterion 3)

EXAMPLE RESPONSES TO ADVANCED-LEVEL CLIENT STATEMENTS FOR EXERCISE 8

Example Response to Advanced Client Statement 1

It sounds like that anger that you are experiencing comes from the belief that they should stick to their word and are bad people for not doing so. (Criterion 1) Is it helping you to believe they should stick to their word when they did not? How does this belief that they should stick to their word and are jerks for not doing so block you from achieving your goals? (Criterion 2) Can you see that holding onto an idea about how they should have acted prevents you from your goal of being annoyed and not angry and therefore better able to express yourself in a constructive manner? (Criterion 3)

Example Response to Advanced Client Statement 2

The depression that you are experiencing may come from these demands about how you should have more of a personality as well as your ratings of your worth or value as a person. (Criterion 1) How does thinking you should have more of a personality and that you are a failure as a person because no one came to your birthday happy hour help you in any way? Are there any negative consequences to these beliefs? (Criterion 2) Can you explain to me how these beliefs that you should have more of a personality as well as that you are a failure as a person because of one event gets in the way of your goal of being sad and not isolating? Do you understand how this belief about you being a failure does not help you to be sad instead of depressed and then impacts your ability to be more social? (Criterion 3)

Example Response to Advanced Client Statement 3

The belief that you should have done more and are a terrible person probably leads to your experiencing guilt. (Criterion 1) Does this belief that you should have done more in her final few months but didn't, and as a result are a terrible person, benefit you in any helpful way? Does this belief create any additional problems for you? (Criterion 2) Do you understand that this expectation of yourself of what you should have done with this family member and that you are a terrible person helps you feel guilt instead of regret? (Criterion 3)

Example Response to Advanced Client Statement 4

The anxiety that you describe sounds like it comes from the beliefs that it would be awful and that you couldn't stand this if you had nothing to say. (Criterion 1) What are the benefits of believing that it would be awful and unbearable? Are there any disadvantages to this belief that you could not handle it and the awfulizing belief? (Criterion 2) Does believing that it would be awful if you had nothing to say help you get you closer to your goal of feeling concerned about this possibility and less likely to cancel? Do you understand that believing that it would be awful and unbearable has a negative impact on you? (Criterion 3)

Example Response to Advanced Client Statement 5

The jealousy that you describe sounds like it comes from the belief that you should be getting these opportunities as well as the fact that it says something about you as a person because you do not. (Criterion 1) Is it helping you or getting in the way to keep holding on to the belief that you should be offered opportunities like your coworker has when that's not what's happening currently and that it reflects on you as a person? (Criterion 2) It sounds like you are demanding that things at work should be fairer and that because you are being overlooked, it means you are incompetent as a person. Do you understand how these beliefs lead to the jealous feelings and do not help you to do your best and obtain some professional opportunities and advancement? (Criterion 3)

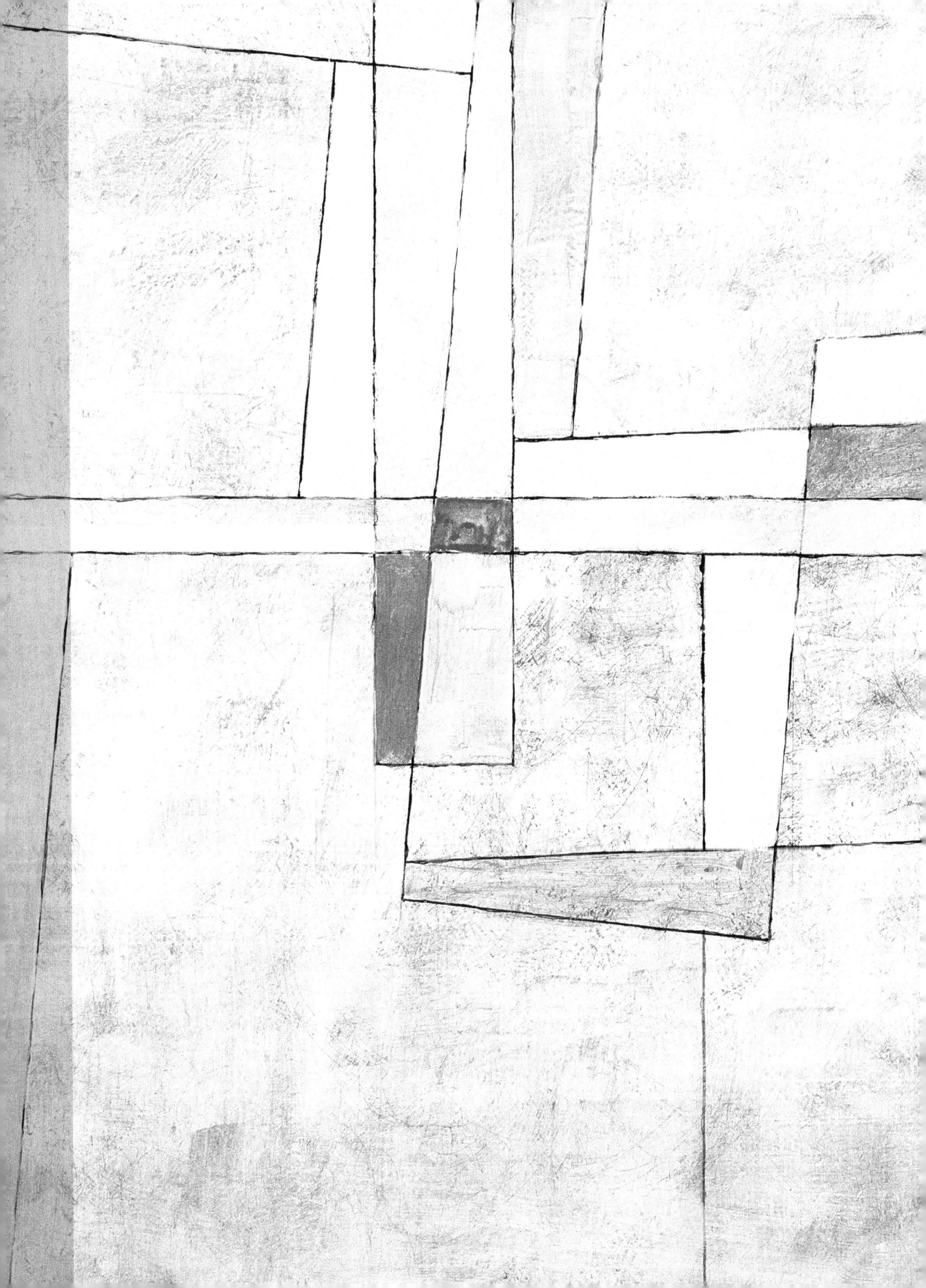

Empirical Disputation of Irrational Beliefs

Preparations for Exercise 9

1. Read the instructions in Chapter 2.

2. Download the Deliberate Practice Reaction Form and the Deliberate Practice Diary Form at https://www.apa.org/pubs/books/deliberate-practice-rational-emotive-behavior-therapy (see the "Clinician and Practitioner Resources" tab; also available in Appendixes A and B, respectively).

Skill Description

Skill Difficulty Level: Advanced

As you learned in the prior exercise, disputing, questioning, or challenging clients' irrational beliefs is an activity that rational emotive behavior therapy (REBT) posits will produce a change in the client's irrational beliefs. An effective REBT clinician will become proficient in applying multiple disputation strategies. One of the core disputation strategies is referred to as an *empirical disputation*. In this, the REBT clinician works with the client to determine whether their irrational beliefs are in fact true, accurate, and consistent with reality. This weakens the strength of their endorsement of the irrational belief by showing that the belief is inconsistent with reality. In so doing, the clinician is challenging the clients' irrational beliefs that lead to maladaptive or unhealthy emotions and dysfunctional behaviors. This skill in this exercise requires the clinician to consider the irrational belief(s) that clients hold about a specific situation and then implement an empirical disputation to help clients give up these beliefs. This entails that clients understand that these beliefs are not supported by empirical reality or are inconsistent with reality.

Very often, irrational beliefs may be implied when the client asks an open-ended question. For example, "What kind of person am I to have done something like that to

https://doi.org/10.1037/0000334-011

Deliberate Practice in Rational Emotive Behavior Therapy, by M. D. Terjesen, K. A. Doyle, R. A. DiGiuseppe, A. Vaz, and T. Rousmaniere

her?" This question implies that because the client behaved a certain way, they may think poorly of themselves; we would categorize this as ratings of worth. A skilled REBT clinician will listen for the implied irrational belief behind a question and propose it as an irrational belief of the client that may be contributing to their emotional and behavioral difficulties. In the advanced client statements, we have added several comments like this to promote trainees' ability to clinically identify an irrational belief of an implied comment or question like that.

Special Considerations for Performing This Exercise

In this exercise, we differentiate the three skill levels (beginner, intermediate, and advanced) in the following manner: For the beginner prompts, clients directly provide one irrational belief; for the intermediate prompts, clients explicitly provide two irrational beliefs; and for the advanced prompts, clients explicitly provide one irrational belief and a second irrational belief that is implied for the clinician to propose what the belief is. We also make this differentiation in skills for the three examples after the skill criteria.

SKILL CRITERIA FOR EXERCISE 9

1. Highlight the main irrational belief presented by the client.
2. Challenge the client's irrational belief using an empirical approach.
3. Check if the client understands that their irrational belief is inconsistent with reality.

Examples of Therapists Using Empirical Disputation of Irrational Beliefs

Example 1

CLIENT: [*angry*] My mother offers her contrary opinion all the time. She shouldn't do this. I would not do this to her, and I ended up yelling at her. Really I don't like feeling this way toward her; I'd prefer to feel really annoyed with her but get along with her better.

THERAPIST: You say that you "don't like feeling this way toward her," and that you want to replace the anger with annoyance or disappointment. In looking at the beliefs that lead to anger, it sounds like you believe that because you do not like her behavior and it is rude, she "should not do this!" (Criterion 1) Where is the empirical evidence for the belief that because it is unpleasant, rude, and you don't like it, "she shouldn't act that way"? In fact, you gave me evidence that she is consistent and acts this way a lot. (Criterion 2) Do you see how these "should" beliefs are not consistent with what you know about her behavior? (Criterion 3)

Example 2

CLIENT: [*anxious*] I am quite sure my boyfriend is going to break up with me. I'm so anxious about this and clingy now, and I can't stand this feeling. I really want to feel concerned instead of anxious. If he did break up with me, it would be terrible!

THERAPIST: It sounds like your belief that "this would be so terrible" is what is leading to you feeling anxious and acting clingy. Since your goal is to replace your anxiety with concern, could we work on disputing or challenging this "awful" type of belief? (Criterion 1) While it most likely would be unpleasant and difficult for you if you broke up, where is the evidence for this belief that "it would be terrible or awful"? (Criterion 2) Do you see how these beliefs about how "terrible" this would be are not consistent with what we know? There really is no proof for this belief. (Criterion 3)

Example 3

CLIENT: [*depressed*] I get asked to go to the gym by my friends all the time and when I have gone, I see they all are in much better shape than I am. No matter how hard I try, I struggle to get more fit. I look at them and then I think I should be able to get in shape. I see myself not just as someone who struggles at the gym, but I also ask myself what's wrong with me and so I've stopped going. Going only makes me feel more depressed. I wish I could go to the gym and be with my friends, and when I see them, I'd rather be sad that it is more of a struggle for me, but not depressed.

THERAPIST: I hear a lot of putting yourself down and a lack of unconditional self-acceptance. This leads to depression and avoidance of going to the gym. (Criterion 1) Let us examine the belief that "I am such a failure as a person." I understand why you want to get more fit, but where is the evidence for the belief that you are a failure as a person—that is you fail at everything—for not meeting your goal of getting more fit? (Criterion 2) Do you understand that this belief is not consistent with what we know to be true? (Criterion 3)

INSTRUCTIONS FOR EXERCISE 9

Step 1: Role-Play and Feedback

- The client says the first beginner client statement. The therapist **improvises** a response based on the skill criteria.
- The trainer (or if not available, the client) provides **brief** feedback based on the skill criteria.
- The client then repeats the same statement, and the therapist again improvises a response. The trainer (or client) again provides brief feedback.

Step 2: Repeat

- Repeat Step 1 for all the statements **in the current difficulty level** (beginner, intermediate, or advanced).

Step 3: Assess and Adjust Difficulty

- The therapist completes the Deliberate Practice Reaction Form (see Appendix A) and decides whether to make the exercise easier or harder or to repeat the same difficulty level.

Step 4: Repeat for Approximately 15 Minutes

- Repeat Steps 1 to 3 for at least 15 minutes.
- The trainees then switch therapist and client roles and start over.

> **Now it's your turn! Follow Steps 1 and 2 from the instructions.**

Remember: The goal of the role-play is for trainees to practice improvising responses to the client statements in a manner that (a) uses the skill criteria and (b) feels authentic for the trainee. **Example therapist responses for each client statement are provided at the end of this exercise. Trainees should attempt to improvise their own responses before reading the example responses.**

BEGINNER-LEVEL CLIENT STATEMENTS FOR EXERCISE 9
Beginner Client Statement 1
[Angry] My anger was through the roof, and I freaked out on her when, at the last minute, my boss dropped a bunch of work for me to do that isn't part of my job. She shouldn't assume I'm going to do it because she can't get her other staff to do their jobs. This is so unfair.
Beginner Client Statement 2
[Depressed] I continue to feel depressed when I think about my 30-year loveless relationship. I want to get out, but this is probably the best I'll ever get because, really, I'm inadequate and see myself as worthless. I guess I'm going to stay stuck in this because in the game of life, I am a failure.
Beginner Client Statement 3
[Guilty] Technically, I have not cheated on my partner, but I have formed an emotional connection with someone else. When asked about it, I lie and say it is nothing, but I feel so guilty. I shouldn't be doing this.
Beginner Client Statement 4
[Anxious] I have to go to a wedding without my long-time partner and am so anxious about people coming up to me and asking why I'm there alone. Having to answer that question would be terrible. Even though it's my close friend's wedding and I want to be there, I am thinking about not going.
Beginner Client Statement 5
[Jealous] My girlfriend seems to prefer this other guy's company over mine. I have been nothing but a good, supportive boyfriend, but now it looks like I am an afterthought. I am so jealous. No one should treat someone like that. I want to stay in this relationship, but I want to lose the jealousy.

 Assess and adjust the difficulty before moving to the next difficulty level (see Step 3 in the exercise instructions).

INTERMEDIATE-LEVEL CLIENT STATEMENTS FOR EXERCISE 9

Intermediate Client Statement 1

[Angry] We had all put in an equal amount of money for the investment property initially, but I worked on fixing the place up and put in my own money and time in. Now that we're selling it, they don't want to reimburse me for this. We had a cursing argument that was so heated, it got physical and someone was thrown to the ground. They should reimburse me for the sale, and I can't stand that they're not.

Intermediate Client Statement 2

[Depressed] I exercise, I diet, but no matter what I do, I can't lose weight. I've started questioning why I'm even bothering. You would think with all this effort, it would be just as easy for me to lose weight as others, but it's not. I should be able to accomplish this goal like others can, and if I can't, that would be awful!

Intermediate Client Statement 3

[Guilty] Almost daily, I plant seeds in my colleague and friend's mind that she shouldn't apply for that promotion because I secretly want it. I know I'm acting in my own interests and that I shouldn't be sneaky and try to block her from her goals. I think I'm a horrible person for doing what I'm doing.

Intermediate Client Statement 4

[Anxious] I have this one chance to show my supervisor that I can do this project. However, I am so anxious about failing that I've been avoiding getting started. I want to prove myself and if I don't and I fail at it, it would be awful and the worst thing that has ever happened to me. If I fail, it would also prove I'm totally incompetent.

Intermediate Client Statement 5

[Jealous] Why do my parents see my brother as the golden child and always favor him over me? I should get to be in the spotlight sometimes and get some recognition for my accomplishments. I can't stand that they always overlook me.

 Assess and adjust the difficulty before moving to the next difficulty level (see Step 3 in the exercise instructions).

ADVANCED-LEVEL CLIENT STATEMENTS FOR EXERCISE 9
Advanced Client Statement 1
[Angry] I was told that the promotion was mine. They then went and hired someone with far less experience than I have, and no one could give me a reason. I was so furious that I lost it and began yelling at them in front of other staffers. They should stick to their word! What kind of people do these things?!
Advanced Client Statement 2
[Depressed] I am so depressed. I noticed that once I retired, all the people who I thought were my friends were just coworkers. No one showed up at my birthday happy hour, which confirms I'm a loser. Why don't I have more of a personality so that others would want to hang out with me?
Advanced Client Statement 3
[Guilty] I am left thinking I should have done more for my mother during her final few months, but I didn't. This makes me a terrible person. Every time I think about what I did—or actually, what I didn't do—I feel so guilty. What does that say about me that I didn't do that? I try not to think about her because I feel so guilty.
Advanced Client Statement 4
[Anxious] We haven't spent time together in years, and what if it's awkward? What if I have nothing to say? That would be awful and unbearable. This scenario is not something I am up for. I'm most likely going to cancel.
Advanced Client Statement 5
[Jealous] Every big professional opportunity seems to go to this one coworker. My reviews are good, so I should be offered some of these opportunities too. Maybe I'm incompetent and that's why I keep getting passed over. We used to be close, but now it's every woman for herself!

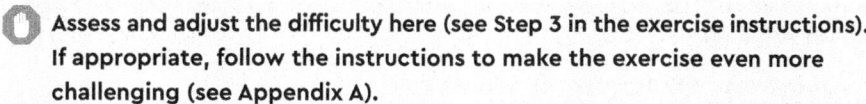 **Assess and adjust the difficulty here (see Step 3 in the exercise instructions). If appropriate, follow the instructions to make the exercise even more challenging (see Appendix A).**

Example Therapist Responses: Empirical Disputation of Irrational Beliefs

Remember: Trainees should attempt to improvise their own responses before reading the example responses. **Do not read the following responses verbatim unless you are having trouble coming up with your own responses!**

EXAMPLE RESPONSES TO BEGINNER-LEVEL CLIENT STATEMENTS FOR EXERCISE 9
Example Response to Beginner Client Statement 1
It sounds like the belief that she "shouldn't do this" is an attitude that leads to your anger. (Criterion 1) Where is the evidence for the belief that "she shouldn't do this"? In fact, you gave me some evidence that she should do it, as she does it quite often. (Criterion 2) Do you understand how these beliefs are actually not true with what we know? (Criterion 3)
Example Response to Beginner Client Statement 2
The depression that you describe sounds like it comes from these negative beliefs you have about yourself and your worth. (Criterion 1) Now, maybe you could have decided to end this relationship earlier. Maybe it would have been better for you to do so, but where is the evidence for the belief that "I am a failure because maybe I made a wrong decision in this one area"? (Criterion 2) Do you understand that those beliefs really have no evidence, and you have no proof to support them? (Criterion 3)
Example Response to Beginner Client Statement 3
You appear to have an irrational belief, "I should not do this to them," that leads to guilt. (Criterion 1) I understand that you wish you didn't do this because you think it was wrong, but what do we know? What is the evidence? You regrettably did do this. So, your belief that you shouldn't do this is inaccurate and not consistent with what we know. (Criterion 2) Do you see how those demanding beliefs really aren't true and have no support? (Criterion 3)
Example Response to Beginner Client Statement 4
Now you said you want to go to the wedding without as much anxiety. To get there, let's examine the belief that "it would be terrible" that leads to anxiety. (Criterion 1) I imagine it would be uncomfortable, but where is the evidence that it would be terrible? Have people asked you already where your partner is? Did you survive? (Criterion 2) If anything, do you understand that the belief really isn't a fact or something we know for certain? (Criterion 3)
Example Response to Beginner Client Statement 5
You have said that you hope to maintain some relationship, but the jealousy interferes with that. It sounds like you are thinking that she "should not treat me this way" and when she does, you make yourself jealous. (Criterion 1) Where is the evidence for this thought that "she shouldn't do this"? In fact, perhaps annoyingly, we have evidence that she does do this regularly. (Criterion 2) If anything, can you see how these beliefs aren't valid and really have no support? (Criterion 3)

EXAMPLE RESPONSES TO INTERMEDIATE-LEVEL CLIENT STATEMENTS FOR EXERCISE 9

Example Response to Intermediate Client Statement 1

It sounds like you are angry that your "partners" really stiffed you on the money you spent upgrading the property. You expressed a demand that they should not have behaved unfairly and stiffed you for the money and another belief, that you can't stand their behavior, is triggering your anger. (Criterion 1) Yes, it is wrong for them not to pay you, but how many times in your life have you noticed that people violate the norms of good behavior and do the wrong thing? Does it happen, even if it's unfortunate? Further, although their behavior may be very wrong, where is the evidence that you can't stand it? (Criterion 2) Do you see that your demand about others' behavior is not consistent with what we know to be true in this situation? Also, the belief about not being able to stand it may not be accurate as well, since you are here telling me about what has occurred. (Criterion 3)

Example Response to Intermediate Client Statement 2

From what you said, I hear that you have the belief that you should be able to lose weight, that it would be awful if you cannot lose weight, and that is what leads you to feel depressed. (Criterion 1) Although it would be disappointing if you are unable to lose weight, would it meet your standard of awful? Just because you really want something, where is it written that you should or must get it? (Criterion 2) Is it realistic to believe that because you struggle with weight loss, that it is awful? Is it consistent with the data that people's demands are always met? (Criterion 3)

Example Response to Intermediate Client Statement 3

The guilt that you describe probably stems from your thinking of yourself as a horrible person along with the idea that you should not behave this way. (Criterion 1) While you are acting badly toward her, that bad behavior is not the sum of your existence and does not make you a horrible person. We all engage in good and bad behaviors. Can you tell me some good things that you do that will challenge the idea that you are a horrible person? And you are saying that you shouldn't do those things, but what do we know: you did. (Criterion 2) Yes, you have behaved poorly toward your colleague. But can you see how it is not consistent with reality to define yourself as only a horrible person for doing this one bad thing? What evidence do you have, besides what is your opinion, that you should not behave badly at times, as opposed to the evidence that you wish you didn't behave badly? (Criterion 3)

Example Response to Intermediate Client Statement 4

The anxiety that you have described is most likely a result of your awfulizing way of thinking about the possibility that you would fail at this project and the belief that this would confirm you are incompetent. (Criterion 1) While if you failed at this project, it would be bad, do you have evidence to support the belief that it would be the worst thing that has ever happened to you and that it would prove that you are totally incompetent? (Criterion 2) Is the idea that failing this one project realistic to be viewed as awful and the worst thing that has ever happened to you? Does it confirm your incompetence? (Criterion 3)

Example Response to Intermediate Client Statement 5

It sounds like your jealousy comes from the belief that they should not always put him in the spotlight and should give you recognition sometimes and that you cannot stand that they do not. (Criterion 1) If they have been rejecting you your whole life, it is likely to happen more, correct? If we had to bet on whether your parents will favor your sibling based on what they have done up to now, where do you place your bet, on how your parents have behaved, or how you demand them to behave? Does the fact that they have done this before and you have frustratingly "survived" show that you can, in fact, handle this—even if it annoys you—when they behave this way again? (Criterion 2) Can you see how those demanding beliefs about their behavior as well as those beliefs that you cannot handle it are not consistent with what is true? (Criterion 3)

EXAMPLE RESPONSES TO ADVANCED-LEVEL CLIENT STATEMENTS FOR EXERCISE 9

Example Response to Advanced Client Statement 1

From what you described, it sounds like the anger you feel comes from a demand about their behavior as well as some ratings of them as people based on what they have done. (Criterion 1) I understand this is unfair to you, but I am wondering where it is written that all people must follow through on their word? Does not doing what one says they will do at times make someone a total jerk as a person? (Criterion 2) Is it consistent with reality that people stick to their word all the time? (Criterion 3)

Example Response to Advanced Client Statement 2

The depression that you describe probably comes from these beliefs that you are a loser and that you should have more of a personality. (Criterion 1) Where is the evidence that you are a failure as a person because no one came to one birthday happy hour? What law exists about what an individual's personality should be? (Criterion 2) And even if you had more of a personality, as you believe you should, is it realistic to think that your coworkers would have shown up? Is it written in the dictionary that the definition of loser is a "failed" birthday happy hour? (Criterion 3)

Example Response to Advanced Client Statement 3

You report that you feel so guilty, and I would hypothesize that feeling comes from the beliefs that you should have done more and are a terrible person. (Criterion 1) Do the Ten Commandments include this belief that you should have done more in her final few months and because you didn't, you're a bad person? Isn't there a saying, "Accept the sinner, not the sin"? (Criterion 2) Is it realistic to believe that you will always do what you should and if you don't, any positive traits you have and behaviors you have done are eliminated? (Criterion 3)

Example Response to Advanced Client Statement 4

The anxiety you describe and your inclination to cancel probably come from the belief that if it was awkward, it would be awful and unbearable. (Criterion 1) Is it really true and consistent with reality that having nothing to say to your friend would be awful and unbearable? Have you stood other times when you didn't add to a conversation? (Criterion 2) Do you understand that you do not have any evidence to support the belief that having nothing to say would be unbearable? (Criterion 3)

Example Response to Advanced Client Statement 5

I can see how continuing to be overlooked for professional opportunities is unfair to you and imagine the jealousy comes from the belief that you "should not" be passed over, and if you are, that means you are "incompetent." (Criterion 1) However, I don't want to seem invalidating, but I wonder where it is written that people should be given opportunities even if they receive good reviews, and that somehow they are totally incompetent if they don't? (Criterion 2) Do you understand that it's not true that only incompetent people are passed over for opportunities, and there might be evidence that many competent people are also passed over and no evidence that they should not be? (Criterion 3)

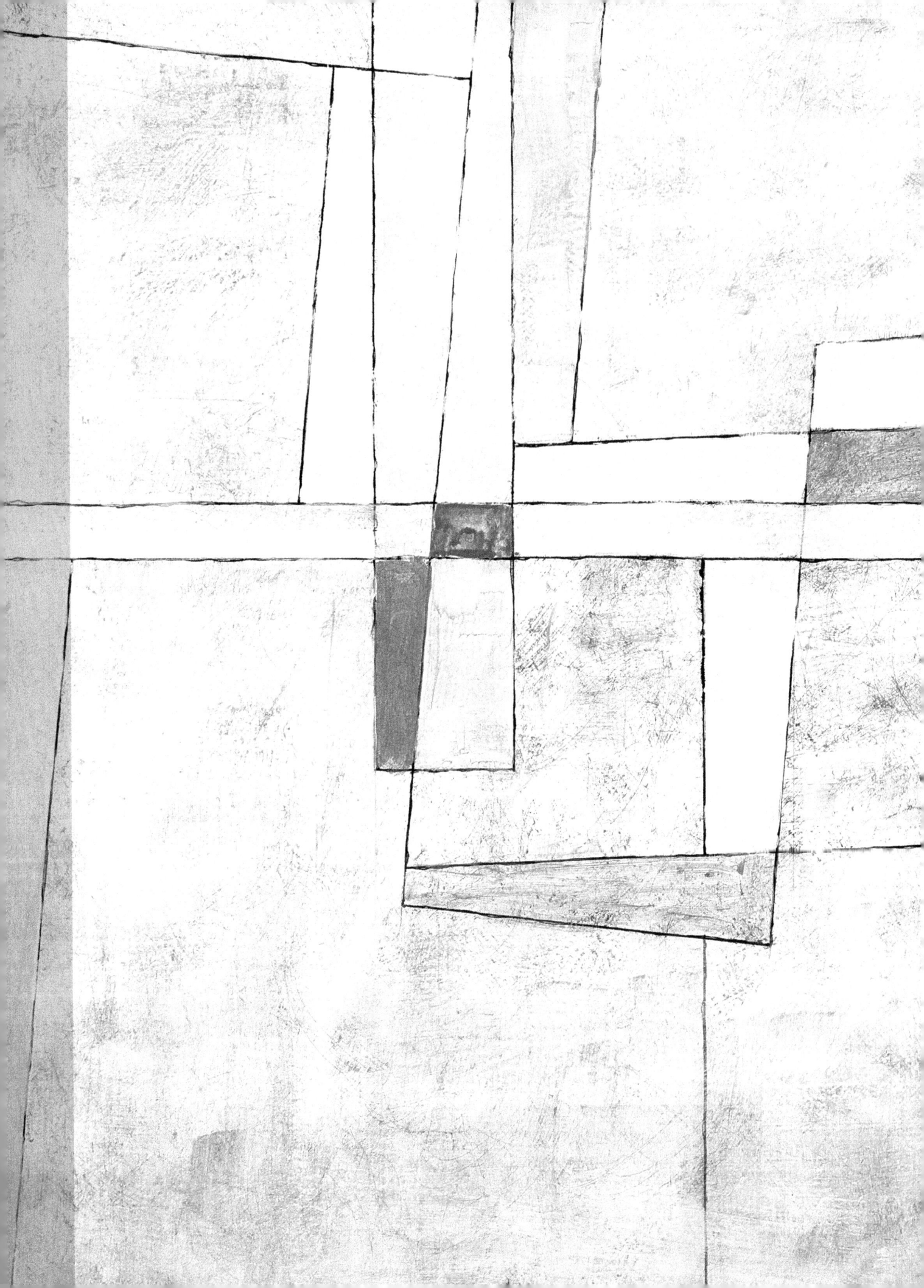

Semantic Disputation of Irrational Beliefs

Preparations for Exercise 10

1. Read the instructions in Chapter 2.

2. Download the Deliberate Practice Reaction Form and the Deliberate Practice Diary Form at https://www.apa.org/pubs/books/deliberate-practice-rational-emotive-behavior-therapy (see the "Clinician and Practitioner Resources" tab; also available in Appendixes A and B, respectively).

Skill Description

Skill Difficulty Level: Advanced

As you learned in the previous two exercises, disputing, questioning, or challenging clients' irrational beliefs are activities that produce a decrease in clients' irrational beliefs and then a change in their unhealthy negative emotions and behaviors. An effective rational emotive behavior therapy (REBT) clinician will become proficient in the application of multiple disputation strategies. One of the core disputation strategies is referred to as a semantic disputation. In this intervention, the REBT clinician works with the client to develop an objective definition (i.e., operationalized in behavioral terms) of the emotionally charged words and phrases that they use that represent their irrational beliefs. That is, an REBT clinician will work with a client to understand the meaning of a word or phrase they use that reflects their irrational beliefs and examine if their use of this word or phrase is consistent with the agreed-on definition. Such discussions help clients see the arbitrary meaning they apply to a word and allows them to assess whether this concept actually applies to the activating event about which they are upset. For example, in clinical work with someone who defines something as "awful" or describes themselves as a "complete loser" or an "idiot," the REBT clinician will dispute

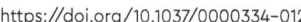

https://doi.org/10.1037/0000334-012

Deliberate Practice in Rational Emotive Behavior Therapy, by M. D. Terjesen, K. A. Doyle, R. A. DiGiuseppe, A. Vaz, and T. Rousmaniere

these beliefs by examining the meaning of the word "awful" (i.e., one of the absolute very worst things that could happen to them), and this could provide them with a reference point for evaluating their view of a specific activating event (e.g., failing a test) as being "awful." This weakens the strength of their endorsement of the irrational belief by showing it to be inconsistent with the meaning of the word. This skill can be done didactically where a definition is provided directly to the client or through a more preferred Socratic approach with more open-ended questions to have the client think about their beliefs and ascertain the client's definition of these beliefs.

This skill requires the clinician to consider and present the irrational belief(s) that clients hold about a specific situation, implement a semantic disputation to help clients give up these beliefs, and ask questions about their belief in a Socratic manner to assist the client in understanding that their definition of their belief is not semantically correct. The clinician does this by asking questions about their belief in a Socratic manner to assist the client in understanding that their definition of their belief is not semantically correct.

Very often irrational beliefs may be implied when the client asks an open-ended question. For example, "What kind of person am I to have done something like that to her?" This question implies that because they behaved a certain way, the client may think poorly of themselves, and we would categorize this as ratings of worth. A good REBT clinician will listen for the implied irrational belief behind a question and propose it as an irrational belief of the client that may be contributing to their emotional and behavioral difficulties. In the advanced client statements, we have added several comments like this to promote the reader's ability to identify clinically an irrational belief of an implied comment or question of this nature.

Special Considerations for Performing This Exercise

In this exercise, we differentiate the three skill levels (beginner, intermediate, and advanced) in the following manner: For the beginner prompts, clients directly provide one irrational belief; for the intermediate-level prompts, clients explicitly provide two irrational beliefs; and for the advanced-level prompts, clients explicitly provide one irrational belief and a second irrational belief that is implied for the clinician to propose what the belief is. We also make this differentiation in skills for the three examples after the skill criteria.

SKILL CRITERIA FOR EXERCISE 10
1. Highlight the main irrational belief presented by the client.
2. Challenge the meaning of the client's irrational belief.
3. Using content from the example, the clinician Socratically challenges the concrete irrational belief.

Examples of Therapists Using Semantic Disputation of Irrational Beliefs

Example 1

CLIENT: [*angry*] My mother offers her contrary opinion all the time. She shouldn't do this. I would not do this to her, and I end up yelling at her. Really, I don't like feeling this way toward her; I'd prefer to feel really annoyed with her but get along with her better.

THERAPIST: You said that you believe that she shouldn't do this, and it sounds like this belief is what leads you to feel angry. (Criterion 1) Let's look at the meaning of the word "should." The word "should" has several meanings in English. It could mean that you think it is advisable that she not do it **or** it could be that it absolutely **must** not happen. The second belief is not true as she does it. When you are most angry, are you applying the latter definition of should? (Criterion 2) When you say, "She shouldn't do this," what do you mean by "should" here? (Criterion 3)

Example 2

CLIENT: [*anxious*] I am quite sure my boyfriend is going to break up with me. I'm so anxious about this and clingy now. I really want to feel concerned instead of anxious. If he did break up with me, it would be terrible!

THERAPIST: You said that if he broke up with you, that would be "terrible" and your future would be "awful"; it sounds like that belief is what makes you feel anxious and behave in a clingy manner. (Criterion 1) While no doubt it would be difficult and upsetting, would this truly meet the criteria or definition of the word "awful"? (Criterion 2) When you say "it would be terrible," what do you mean by the word "terrible"? (Criterion 3)

Example 3

CLIENT: [*depressed*] I get asked to go to the gym by my friends all the time and when I have gone, I see they all are in much better shape than I am. No matter how hard I try, I struggle to get more fit. I look at them and then I think I should be able to get in shape. I see myself not just as someone who struggles at the gym, but I also ask myself what's wrong with me and so I've stopped going. Going only makes me feel more depressed. I wish I could go to the gym and be with my friends, and when I see them, I'd rather be sad that it is more of a struggle for me, but not depressed.

THERAPIST: The depression that you are describing sounds like it comes from the beliefs that you are a failure as a person. (Criterion 1) How does the fact that you struggle more in getting fit make you a "failure" as a person? (Criterion 2) When you say, "I am a failure as a person," what do you mean by "failure"? Is your self-worth defined by your ability to get more fit? (Criterion 3)

INSTRUCTIONS FOR EXERCISE 10

Step 1: Role-Play and Feedback

- The client says the first beginner client statement. The therapist **improvises** a response based on the skill criteria.
- The trainer (or, if not available, the client) provides **brief** feedback based on the skill criteria.
- The client then repeats the same statement, and the therapist again improvises a response. The trainer (or client) again provides brief feedback.

Step 2: Repeat

- Repeat Step 1 for all the statements **in the current difficulty level** (beginner, intermediate, or advanced).

Step 3: Assess and Adjust Difficulty

- The therapist completes the Deliberate Practice Reaction Form (see Appendix A) and decides whether to make the exercise easier or harder or to repeat the same difficulty level.

Step 4: Repeat for Approximately 15 Minutes

- Repeat Steps 1 to 3 for at least 15 minutes.
- The trainees then switch therapist and client roles and start over.

Now it's your turn! Follow Steps 1 and 2 from the instructions.

Remember: The goal of the role-play is for trainees to practice improvising responses to the client statements in a manner that (a) uses the skill criteria and (b) feels authentic for the trainee. **Example therapist responses for each client statement are provided at the end of this exercise. Trainees should attempt to improvise their own responses before reading the example responses.**

BEGINNER-LEVEL CLIENT STATEMENTS FOR EXERCISE 10
Beginner Client Statement 1
[Angry] My anger was through the roof, and I freaked out on her when, at the last minute, my boss dropped a bunch of work for me to do that isn't part of my job. She shouldn't assume I'm going to do it because she can't get her other staff to do their jobs. This is so unfair.
Beginner Client Statement 2
[Depressed] I continue to feel depressed when I think about my 30-year loveless relationship. I want to get out, but this is probably the best I'll ever get because, really, I'm inadequate and see myself as worthless. I guess I'm going to stay stuck in this because in the game of life, I am a failure.
Beginner Client Statement 3
[Guilty] Technically, I have not cheated on my partner, but I have formed an emotional connection with someone else. When asked about it, I lie and say it is nothing, but I feel so guilty. I shouldn't be doing this.
Beginner Client Statement 4
[Anxious] I have to go to a wedding without my long-time partner and am so anxious about people coming up to me and asking why I'm there alone. Having to answer that question would be terrible. Even though it's my close friend's wedding and I want to be there, I am thinking about not going.
Beginner Client Statement 5
[Jealous] My girlfriend seems to prefer this other guy's company over mine. I have been nothing but a good, supportive boyfriend, but now it looks like I am an afterthought. I am so jealous. No one should treat someone like that. I want to stay in this relationship, but I want to lose the jealousy.

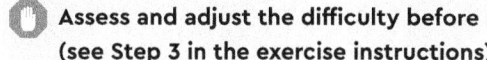 **Assess and adjust the difficulty before moving to the next difficulty level (see Step 3 in the exercise instructions).**

INTERMEDIATE-LEVEL CLIENT STATEMENTS FOR EXERCISE 10
Intermediate Client Statement 1
[Angry] We had all put in an equal amount of money for the investment property initially, but I worked on fixing the place up and put in my own money and time. Now that we're selling it, they don't want to reimburse me for this. We had a cursing argument that was so heated, and it got physical and someone was thrown to the ground. They should reimburse me for the sale, and I can't stand that they're not.
Intermediate Client Statement 2
[Depressed] I exercise, I diet, but no matter what I do, I can't lose weight. I've started questioning why I'm even bothering. You would think with all this effort it would be just as easy for me to lose weight as others, but it's not. It just proves what a loser I am.
Intermediate Client Statement 3
[Guilty] Almost daily, I plant seeds in my colleague and friend's mind that she shouldn't apply for that promotion because I secretly want it. I know I'm acting in my own interests and I know I shouldn't be sneaky and try to block her from her goals. I think I'm a horrible person for doing what I'm doing.
Intermediate Client Statement 4
[Anxious] I have this one chance to show my supervisor that I can do this project. However, I am so anxious about failing that I've been avoiding getting started. I want to prove myself and if I don't and I fail at it, it would be awful and the worst thing that has ever happened to me. If I fail, it would also prove I'm totally incompetent.
Intermediate Client Statement 5
[Jealous] Why do my parents see my brother as the golden child and always favor him over me? I should get to be in the spotlight sometimes and get some recognition for my accomplishments. I'm clearly not good enough in my parents' eyes.

 Assess and adjust the difficulty before moving to the next difficulty level (see Step 3 in the exercise instructions).

ADVANCED-LEVEL CLIENT STATEMENTS FOR EXERCISE 10

Advanced Client Statement 1

[Angry] I was told that the promotion was mine. They then went and hired someone with far less experience than I have, and no one could give me a reason. I was so furious that I lost it and began yelling at them in front of other staffers. They should stick to their word! What kind of people do these things?!

Advanced Client Statement 2

[Depressed] I am so depressed. I noticed that once I retired, all the people who I thought were my friends were just coworkers. No one showed up at my birthday happy hour, which confirms I'm a loser. Why don't I have more of a personality so that others would want to hang out with me?

Advanced Client Statement 3

[Guilty] I am left thinking I should have done more for my mother during her final few months, but I didn't. This makes me a terrible person. Every time I think about what I did—or actually, what I didn't do—I feel so guilty. What does that say about me that I didn't do that? I try not to think about her because I feel so guilty.

Advanced Client Statement 4

[Anxious] We haven't spent time together in years, and what if it's awkward? What if I have nothing to say? That would be awful and unbearable. This scenario is not something I am up for. I'm most likely going to cancel.

Advanced Client Statement 5

[Jealous] Every big professional opportunity seems to go to this one coworker. My reviews are good, so I should be offered some of these opportunities too. Maybe I'm incompetent and that's why I keep getting passed over. We used to be close, but now it's every woman for herself!

🔘 **Assess and adjust the difficulty here (see Step 3 in the exercise instructions). If appropriate, follow the instructions to make the exercise even more challenging (see Appendix A).**

Example Therapist Responses: Semantic Disputation of Irrational Beliefs

Remember: Trainees should attempt to improvise their own responses before reading the example responses. **Do not read the following responses verbatim unless you are having trouble coming up with your own responses!**

EXAMPLE RESPONSES TO BEGINNER-LEVEL CLIENT STATEMENTS FOR EXERCISE 10
Example Response to Beginner Client Statement 1
You said that "she shouldn't assume I'm going to do it" and those beliefs are probably what leads you to feel angry. (Criterion 1) While I imagine it is quite annoying and frustrating, the words "should not" imply the belief that they "have not," "must not," or "need not" to do this. Is this idea truly a have to, must, or need? (Criterion 2) When you say, "She shouldn't do that behavior," what do you mean by that? That you literally need that this not to occur for survival purposes? (Criterion 3)
Example Response to Beginner Client Statement 2
It sounds like you feel depressed when you believe that you are a failure in life because of the status of your relationship. (Criterion 1) Is the idea that "I am a failure because of my relationship" accurate? A complete failure fails—always. (Criterion 2) When you say that you are "inadequate" and "worthless," what do you mean by "inadequate" and "worthless"? What do you mean by saying your worth and value as a human being is contingent on how loving your 30-year-long relationship is? (Criterion 3)
Example Response to Beginner Client Statement 3
While you might think your behavior is wrong, and let's say it is, you say that you think that "you shouldn't be doing this," and that appears to lead to you feeling guilty. (Criterion 1) If we define "shoulds" as essentials or absolute "have-tos," does your "should" meet the criteria or definition of the word? Are you free to make bad choices and not always do the right thing, like you are demanding of yourself? (Criterion 2) When you say "I shouldn't," what exactly do you mean by that? (Criterion 3)
Example Response to Beginner Client Statement 4
You said that if they judged you, it would be terrible, and I assume that is what leads to you feel anxious and consider not going. (Criterion 1) While we don't know that they will judge you, if this did happen, would this be something completely awful? (Criterion 2) When you say "It would be terrible," what do you mean by that? That it would be the worst thing that could ever happen to you? (Criterion 3)
Example Response to Beginner Client Statement 5
"Should" implies that she "needs" to act this way, and for you, it sounds like this leads you to being jealous. (Criterion 1) Needs by definition are things that are essential for survival. Is how you want her to treat you really a need? Does it meet the definition that without it, you would cease to exist? (Criterion 2) When you say "should," what do you mean by the word "should"? (Criterion 3)

EXAMPLE RESPONSES TO INTERMEDIATE-LEVEL CLIENT STATEMENTS FOR EXERCISE 10

Example Response to Intermediate Client Statement 1

It sounds like the demand that they should reimburse you and you can't stand that they haven't makes you angry. (Criterion 1) I know you want this to happen, but if this truly is a "should" and it must happen, then it would have. While their behavior is wrong, is it a "have-to"? If you really could not stand this reality of not being reimbursed, would you be alive and talking to me about it? (Criterion 2) What do you mean when you believe that they should do the right thing? What are the things in life that we really can't stand? (Criterion 3)

Example Response to Intermediate Client Statement 2

From what I hear, you have two beliefs that are bound to leave you depressed: One is that you should be able to lose weight like others do, and the other is that you believe it would be awful if you cannot. (Criterion 1) If we examine what should happen in this world according to laws of physics, does your "should" match that? If you are unable to lose weight like your friends, would it truly be the end of the world and nothing worse could happen? (Criterion 2) How do you define "should"? Is "should" different from "want"? The word "awful" means a lot of things to different people. What do you mean when you say it would be "awful" if you didn't achieve this weight goal? (Criterion 3)

Example Response to Intermediate Client Statement 3

The guilt that you have described sounds like it comes from some beliefs about yourself, like I am a horrible person, and I shouldn't be acting this way. (Criterion 1) Although you may be acting badly toward her, how does that one bad behavior equal the sum of your existence? The rigidly held belief of should implies that whatever we are demanding happen is a necessity, like the needs for water, air, or food. Is that behavior here a necessity? (Criterion 2) Does it follow that your bad behavior toward her defines yourself and your worth? (Criterion 3) You also seem to be demanding that you should not be acting sneaky. Based on this understanding of the definition of a dogmatic "should," how would you define your behavior relative to this definition? (Criterion 3)

Example Response to Intermediate Client Statement 4

What I am hearing is that the anxiety you experience comes from thinking that if you fail, it would be awful and would prove you're totally incompetent. (Criterion 1) There is no doubt that it would be disappointing if you failed this project, but let's look at your use of the word "awful." Awful implies beyond bad. Would this potential outcome meet that definition? If you fail at this one project, how does that failing make you totally incompetent as a person? (Criterion 2) What things would we get some near unanimity among others that would meet an awful classification? Would this be on that list? By definition, wouldn't you need to be incompetent at everything you do to prove you are an incompetent person? (Criterion 3)

Example Response to Intermediate Client Statement 5

It sounds like you are believing that your parents "should" recognize your accomplishments and they don't; plus, you have a belief that you can't stand always being overlooked by them, and that's when you experience jealousy. (Criterion 1) The word "should" implies that it is a need, must, or have-to. Given this, does your "should" about recognition meet that definition? The idea "I can't stand that they always overlook me" would imply that you wouldn't be alive to tell me about this. (Criterion 2) Let's discuss what you mean by "should" and "I can't stand" and see whether these ideas meet your definitions. (Criterion 3)

EXAMPLE RESPONSES TO ADVANCED-LEVEL CLIENT STATEMENTS FOR EXERCISE 10

Example Response to Advanced Client Statement 1

The emotion of anger and the behaviors that you describe sound like they may come from a demand you make about their behavior and some other-condemnation beliefs about them. (Criterion 1) If something "should" happen, by definition, it would happen. Can you see how you're giving them a global rating because they did not follow your demands of what should happen? (Criterion 2) Saying they "should" have acted in a certain way is akin to saying they "need" to act in a certain way. Does anyone really need to act in a certain way? Generally speaking, are there things that we all sometimes don't do that we should? If you act differently than someone else, does that define you globally as a bad person? (Criterion 3)

Example Response to Advanced Client Statement 2

When you describe being depressed, that feeling may derive from the belief that you should have more of a personality and because you believe you don't, are a loser. (Criterion 1) Can you see that if something should happen, it actually would—like a pencil dropping to the floor because of gravity? And a loser is someone who loses 100% of the time—past, present, and future. Do you meet this criterion? (Criterion 2) Do you believe having more of a personality is highly desirable or a dogmatic demand? How does the fact that others did not attend a social event make you a total failure as a person? What is your definition of being a total failure look like? (Criterion 3)

Example Response to Advanced Client Statement 3

You describe feeling very guilty, and from what I am hearing, these feelings stem from the idea that you are a terrible person because you should have done more for your mother. (Criterion 1) How many bad things does a person have to do to be a totally bad person? Can you see how saying you should have done more would mean that you would have done more? (Criterion 2) Can you tell me any good things you have done in the past? Can you accurately define yourself as totally good or totally bad? In your mind, what is the difference between wanting versus expecting or demanding something? (Criterion 3)

Example Response to Advanced Client Statement 4

The anxiety you describe and the fact that you are considering canceling, most likely is a result of your thinking it may be awkward and that would be terrible and that you couldn't tolerate the interaction being awkward. (Criterion 1) Awful is 101% bad, and it could never be worse. Is it the worst thing in the world if it was awkward, even if very awkward? Do you really believe you would die from an awkward interaction? (Criterion 2) Can you think of any other things in your life that have happened or could happen that could be worse than your having an awkward interaction with your friend? What is your definition of something being awful? Can you tell me things in life that are actually truly intolerable or unbearable for anyone to deal with? Would this situation meet that criterion? (Criterion 3)

Example Response to Advanced Client Statement 5

The jealousy you describe may come from the beliefs that you have about yourself being an incompetent person and that you should be offered this position. (Criterion 1) Being an incompetent person means you are incompetent at everything you do. Can you honestly tell me you are incompetent at everything you do? And I know that you want these opportunities, but if something "should" happen, it would. (Criterion 2) Can you think of another way of defining yourself when you get passed over for a professional opportunity that doesn't define you as completely incompetent as a person? Can you explain the difference between **wanting** to get some professional opportunities and **demanding** that you get them? (Criterion 3)

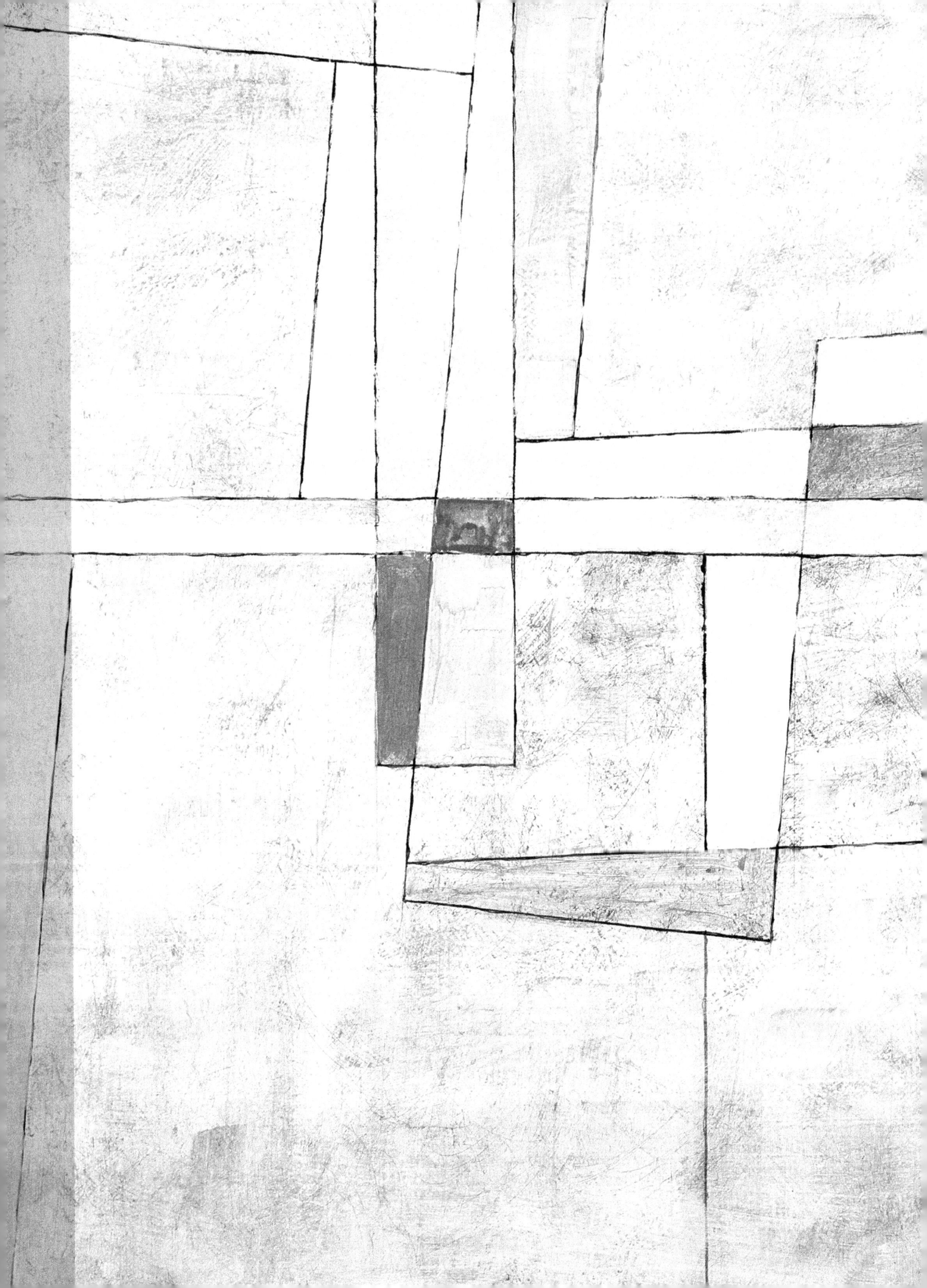

Constructing Full Rational Alternative Beliefs to Replace Irrational Beliefs

Preparations for Exercise 11

1. Read the instructions in Chapter 2.

2. Download the Deliberate Practice Reaction Form and the Deliberate Practice Diary Form at https://www.apa.org/pubs/books/deliberate-practice-rational-emotive-behavior-therapy (see the "Clinician and Practitioner Resources" tab; also available in Appendixes A and B, respectively).

Skill Description

Skill Difficulty Level: Advanced

As you have learned thus far, rational emotive behavior therapy (REBT) practitioners teach clients many skills to achieve their emotional and behavioral goals. At this point, we have presented exercises about providing psychoeducation about REBT, prioritizing irrational beliefs, teaching the belief–consequence (B-C) connection, and restructuring (challenging) irrational beliefs with three types of disputes. The next skill focuses on constructing full rational alternative beliefs (FRABs) that are a functional alternative to the irrational beliefs that clients can learn in session. We caution that it is important the client learn and can apply the skills taught in previous exercises before moving to the construction of FRABs with the client. If the practitioner moves too quickly to generating rational alternative beliefs without the foundational skills taught, demonstrated, and practiced up until this point, clients might often be misled into thinking that all that is required to feel better emotionally and behave more adaptively is "simply" to replace their irrational beliefs with rational beliefs. A common response from clients when they are being taught how to construct FRABs to their current irrational beliefs is the following: "So all I have to do is tell myself this, and I won't feel angry/depressed/guilty, etc.?"

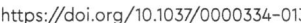

https://doi.org/10.1037/0000334-013

Deliberate Practice in Rational Emotive Behavior Therapy, by M. D. Terjesen, K. A. Doyle, R. A. DiGiuseppe, A. Vaz, and T. Rousmaniere

REBT practitioners are encouraged to explain to their clients that they are experiencing emotional and behavioral disturbance because they have rehearsed the irrational beliefs for some time and probably have done so with force or energy. Therefore, to make a philosophical shift in one's belief system, it is important to stress to clients that in addition to challenging the irrational beliefs, they might require consistent rehearsal with strong force of the new full rational alternative beliefs to strengthen their conviction in this new belief system.

To help therapists learn to construct a FRAB, we offer some guidelines. A FRAB always includes either the acceptance of reality as it is or a rational evaluation statement. It will also include a negation of the irrational demand or evaluation. This results in FRABs always being compound sentences. If you have a short, one-phrase sentence, the belief expressed might be rational, but it is not a FRAB.

We think it would be helpful to provide examples of FRABs for the four major irrational beliefs. The FRAB counterpart of a demanding irrational belief is a preference that both endorses a rational belief and negates the irrational belief. For example, if an irrational belief states, "I want X to respect me, therefore X must (should, ought to, or have to) respect me," the rational belief (but not the FRAB) would be "I want and prefer that X respects me." With such a rationally worded sentence, the client often does not give up their irrational belief. However, this rational preference belief states just the preference and does not provide a negation of the "must." As a result, it might not counter the irrational "must." A full rational alternative belief includes not only the rational references but also the counter of the irrational element of the irrational idea. Thus, the FRAB for the irrational belief in this paragraph would be "I want X to respect me, and I recognize that, even though I want X to respect me, X does not have to respect me."

Imagine using the same principles to construct the full rational alternative belief for an awfulizing irrational belief, such as "It is awful that X does not respect me." The FRAB would acknowledge the realistic negative appraisal of the event and negate the awfulness. The FRAB would be "It is bad and disappointing that X does not respect me, but even though it is bad, it is not awful."

Using the same strategy, we can create a full rational alternative belief for frustration intolerance. Rational frustration tolerance acknowledges that a situation is difficult and challenging, but not too difficult. Using the same activating event, the following could be the full rational alternative: "It is difficult to live with the fact that X does not respect me; however, even though it is difficult, I can stand it."

We can also create FRABs for irrational beliefs about global worth of human beings. The opposite of condemnation of the self or others would endorse self or other acceptance. A self-condemnation irrational belief about the same activating event (feeling disrespected) might be "I must be a real loser and a worthless person if X doesn't respect me." Here, the FRAB could be "I am disappointed that X doesn't respect me, but I can accept myself because it does not make me less of a person or a loser because X does not respect me." An irrational global evaluation of another person might be "X is a pompous loser if X does not respect me." The FRAB here could be "I am disappointed that X does not respect me, but I can accept that he is a person who has worth and not a loser even if he does not respect me."

A common error evidenced in implementing this skill involves the REBT practitioner failing to generate a complete, or full, rational alternative that negates the current irrational belief(s) their client espouses. This error results in clients not relinquishing their irrational belief(s) and thereby continuing to experience disturbance. For example, if the irrational belief is "Other people must respect me," and the practitioner proposes the alternative of "I want people to respect me," room is left for the client to "sneak" back in a must, by saying, "I want people to respect me, as they must!" The solution to this problem is to construct the rational belief to be "I want people to respect me, and I recognize that even though I want it, they do not have to respect me."

Irrational beliefs are highly correlated with each another, and it is common for clients to endorse multiple irrational beliefs, such as a demandingness, an awfulizing, and a frustration intolerance belief about their activating events. A common mistake REBT practitioners make involves an attempt to construct a rational alternative that does not directly address or counter the irrational belief they have been discussing because they have gone back and forth discussing multiple irrational beliefs. Thus, they start challenging one irrational belief but provide the FRAB for another irrational belief that the client endorses. That is, they construct a belief that might be rational but is not the rational alternative to the irrational belief endorsed by the client that they have been disputing. As an example, suppose a client believes several IBs about failing, and one is "It would be awful if I failed." The client or therapist could generate a FRAB such as "I can stand it if I fail." The irrational belief they have been addressing is about awfulizing, and the rational alternative is about frustration tolerance, which is not consistent with that awfulizing belief. It is important that clinicians be mindful that the new rational belief that they generate be consistent and a functional alternative to the irrational belief that has been the topic of the discussions. The rational belief that "I can stand it if I fail" might be rational and might be helpful, but it does not follow from the discussion the therapist and client have just had about awfulizing beliefs. The FRAB for the irrational belief "It would be awful if I failed" would be "It would be bad if I failed, but not awful or terrible." This allows the clinician to be consistent with the belief domain and validate the aversive nature of the adversity without validating the awfulizing component.

Special Considerations for Performing This Exercise

We have differentiated the various skill levels (beginner, intermediate, and advanced) by presenting one irrational belief, then two, and, by the advanced skill level, three irrational beliefs. You should keep in mind that the goal when constructing the alternative full rational belief(s) is to ensure that you (a) address the accurate irrational belief(s) the client is identifying that results in emotional and/or behavioral disturbance and (b) generate a full rational belief that does not allow the client any opportunity to continue holding on to the irrational belief to assist the client in achieving their emotional and behavioral goals. When responding to the vignettes, you want to assume that the aforementioned prerequisite skills have been taught and mastered by the client.

SKILL CRITERIA FOR EXERCISE 11
1. Formulate the full alternative rational belief(s).
2. Check if the client sees how the new full alternative rational belief(s) result in a healthy negative emotion and adaptive behavior.

Examples of Therapists Constructing Full Rational Alternative Beliefs to Replace Irrational Beliefs

Example 1

CLIENT: [*angry*] I show up earlier than everyone else for work. I leave after everyone else and spend nights and weekends addressing work-related issues. I realize that some of this is self-inflicted, but other aspects are not, and people assume I am available 24 hours a day, 7 days a week for this job. I love my job, but I realize that given the history and current circumstances, I have to set boundaries. I'm so angry with myself because I know what I should be doing, and for some reason I'm not doing it. I know those angry thoughts at myself don't make sense, but I believe that I should draw a line in the sand and tell them no, but I don't. I give in, respond, and then get really angry at myself for doing so, and just end up ruminating. I don't want to keep feeling angry with my behavior, but I also want to start setting some boundaries. If I felt more annoyed with myself, I think I could set those boundaries and not waste whatever personal time I have left doing things I enjoy rather than ruminating.

THERAPIST: You say that your anger stems from the demand that you "should" be setting boundaries around work but aren't. Having already established that those demands aren't helping you, I wonder if you replaced that unhealthy demand with a more flexible belief, such as "I really want to set boundaries with work, but there is no law that says I must." (Criterion 1) You might achieve your goal of feeling annoyed when you don't set a boundary, but also not waste your time ruminating. Do you see how those healthier beliefs and the emotion of annoyance may also help you to problem solve ways of "drawing a line in the sand" as you stated? (Criterion 2)

Example 2

CLIENT: [*anxious*] I really like this guy at work, and we have some good witty banter. We joke around a lot, and it seems like there is some connection there between us. It's been 5 months that this has been going on, but he hasn't asked me out. At this point, I want to ask him out to see if there is something there, but I stop myself because I'm so anxious. I think if I ask him out and he says no, that would be horrible, and I couldn't stand being around him at work. I know those beliefs got in the way of my acting. I wish I could feel concern about the possibility of being rejected and still go for it.

THERAPIST: From what you are saying, your anxiety is coming from the irrational beliefs that if you ask him out and get rejected, it would be horrible and then you couldn't stand being around him at work. As you pointed out, those beliefs get in the way of you doing something. We could replace those irrational beliefs with healthier, alternative rational ones, such as "If I get rejected that would be very bad, but not horrible" and "I would not like being around him at work if he rejected me, but even though I would not like it, I certainly could stand it." (Criterion 1) If you really believed these alternative ideas, you could probably experience a healthy concern about his response, and if it did not turn out as you hoped, you might feel uncomfortable around him at work, but you could survive it. Does that make sense? (Criterion 2)

Example 3

CLIENT: [*depressed*] I'm feeling really depressed lately. Ever since the start of the pandemic, my social life is down the drain. I have really tried hard like we talked about to get myself out there to meet someone. But now it seems like people aren't really going out to meet others. I keep thinking, "I should not be in this situation at this stage of my life" and "I'm such a loser because I am." I know that those beliefs only create depression and withdrawal, and as we talked about, they don't make sense or help me reach my goals. I don't want to feel depressed about this, and I want to keep persevering. I guess if I felt sad or disappointed about the current situation, I might be more motivated to push through this challenge.

THERAPIST: So, you see how telling yourself that you "should not" be in this situation, and you're a loser because you are, leads you to feel depressed and to withdraw. I suggest that we replace those irrational, unhelpful beliefs with healthier more adaptive ones. How about replacing them with beliefs such as "I really wish I wasn't in this situation at this stage of my life, but there is no reason I must get what I wish" and "Even though I do not like being in this situation, it does not define me as a total loser as a person"? (Criterion 1) If you were to start believing those rational beliefs in your gut, can you see that you could probably feel, let's say, sad or disappointed at your current situation but not depressed? Would you be more likely to continue pushing through rather than withdrawing? (Criterion 2)

INSTRUCTIONS FOR EXERCISE 11

Step 1: Role-Play and Feedback

- The client says the first beginner client statement. The therapist **improvises** a response based on the skill criteria.
- The trainer (or if not available, the client) provides **brief** feedback based on the skill criteria.
- The client then repeats the same statement, and the therapist again improvises a response. The trainer (or client) again provides brief feedback.

Step 2: Repeat

- Repeat Step 1 for all the statements **in the current difficulty level** (beginner, intermediate, or advanced).

Step 3: Assess and Adjust Difficulty

- The therapist completes the Deliberate Practice Reaction Form (see Appendix A) and decides whether to make the exercise easier or harder or to repeat the same difficulty level.

Step 4: Repeat for Approximately 15 Minutes

- Repeat Steps 1 to 3 for at least 15 minutes.
- The trainees then switch therapist and client roles and start over.

> **Now it's your turn! Follow Steps 1 and 2 from the instructions.**

Remember: The goal of the role-play is for trainees to practice improvising responses to the client statements in a manner that (a) uses the skill criteria and (b) feels authentic for the trainee. **Example therapist responses for each client statement are provided at the end of this exercise. Trainees should attempt to improvise their own responses before reading the example responses.**

BEGINNER-LEVEL CLIENT STATEMENTS FOR EXERCISE 11
Beginner Client Statement 1
[Angry] I must help all my clients get better. If I don't, I'll feel angry at myself and ruminate. I now see how this isn't helpful, but honestly, I'm not sure what else to think.
Beginner Client Statement 2
[Depressed] If I get rejected, that proves I'm an inadequate person. That will make me so depressed, and I'll end up isolating myself again. I know that is just one aspect of who I am, but what can I tell myself so I don't feel depressed and then isolate? I'm so sick of this.
Beginner Client Statement 3
[Guilty] I shouldn't have lied to my friend. I feel guilty, and now I'm avoiding her. I don't want to avoid her, and even though I know thinking this way isn't helpful, I can't get away from this guilt.
Beginner Client Statement 4
[Anxious] Being disapproved of is terrible! I'm so anxious about the meeting that I'm thinking of calling out sick. You've shown me how thinking this way is not helpful; how else can I think?
Beginner Client Statement 5
[Jealous] He should pay more attention to me than to her. I'm jealous that he picks her over me, and I keep checking his phone to see how long they speak each day. Yes, as we've discussed, I know this jealousy doesn't help, and I know I'm only making matters worse by believing this, but I don't see a different way of looking at it.

🛑 **Assess and adjust the difficulty before moving to the next difficulty level (see Step 3 in the exercise instructions).**

INTERMEDIATE-LEVEL CLIENT STATEMENTS FOR EXERCISE 11
Intermediate Client Statement 1
[Angry] I'm so angry. I should have gotten a raise, and my boss is a jerk for overlooking me. I agree that these beliefs don't make me feel better, and I'm willing to try another way of thinking, but I just can't seem to come up with anything.
Intermediate Client Statement 2
[Depressed] I really believe that I should have more social plans and because I don't, it means I'm a failure. I feel depressed, which only makes me want to avoid people. I now see how my depression is related to my belief about myself and my subsequent avoidance. I get that. I just can't come up with anything different to believe instead.
Intermediate Client Statement 3
[Guilty] I should call my mother more, and because I don't, I'm a bad person. Now with all this guilt, I'm avoiding her calls. Sure, as we've discussed avoiding her calls because of my "should" and my guilt is only making my situation worse. What can I tell myself to pick up the stupid phone and just face her?
Intermediate Client Statement 4
[Anxious] I must not make a mistake during my presentation, and if I do, it would be horrible! I'm so anxious that I'm spending all my time preparing and not getting any of my other work done. I have no time to myself because of all this horribilizing and overpreparing. From our conversations, I see that. How do I stop this? What do I tell myself instead?
Intermediate Client Statement 5
[Jealous] My boyfriend must show me that he loves me, and if he doesn't, that proves I'm a worthless person. My jealousy is making me into a nag. I don't want to be a nag—I want a healthy relationship. I see my beliefs are problematic. Please, what can I say to myself not to be jealous and not to be a nag?

 Assess and adjust the difficulty before moving to the next difficulty level (see Step 3 in the exercise instructions).

ADVANCED-LEVEL CLIENT STATEMENTS FOR EXERCISE 11
Advanced Client Statement 1
[Angry] People should respect me, and I can't stand it when they don't. They really are incompetent morons. I'm angry all the time and have become very argumentative with people. I hate being angry and argumentative. I know I have to change my views of what's going on and can't change them. What do you suggest?
Advanced Client Statement 2
[Depressed] I shouldn't have had so much loss in my life. It's unbearable and truly awful. I play these losses over and over again in my head and think how awful my life is and feel such depression. Thinking this way isn't going to change anything. I know I have to change my thinking, but I'm finding it hard what to tell myself when I have those moments of rumination. Do you have any suggestions?
Advanced Client Statement 3
[Guilty] I should have gone to my parents' anniversary party, and I didn't, which makes me a really bad person. I just can't stand the idea of facing them. I feel so guilty about this, and have avoided calling them. I'm tired of thinking this way and then continuing to act poorly. I have to get out of this unhealthy cycle. What do you suggest I should think instead?
Advanced Client Statement 4
[Anxious] I have to make a good impression with my coworkers and couldn't tolerate it if I don't. If they have a poor opinion of me, that proves I'm a total failure. My anxiety is through the roof, and I've started acting weird around them when I think this way. I'm at a loss. Any help in a different way of thinking would be appreciated.
Advanced Client Statement 5
[Jealous] He should shower me with attention and love, and if he doesn't, that would be awful and truly show just how worthless of a human being I am. I'm jealous of everyone he talks to and have become so needy with him. I see what you're saying about how these beliefs are only getting in my way. I don't know where to start to change things.

> **Assess and adjust the difficulty here (see Step 3 in the exercise instructions). If appropriate, follow the instructions to make the exercise even more challenging (see Appendix A).**

Example Therapist Responses: Constructing Full Rational Alternative Beliefs to Replace Irrational Beliefs

Remember: Trainees should attempt to improvise their own responses before reading the example responses. **Do not read the following responses verbatim unless you are having trouble coming up with your own responses!**

EXAMPLE RESPONSES TO BEGINNER-LEVEL CLIENT STATEMENTS FOR EXERCISE 11
Example Response to Beginner Client Statement 1
What if instead you started thinking, "I really want to help all of my clients get better, but there's no reason I absolutely must do so"? (Criterion 1) Can you see if you really believed this new, healthier alternative, you would not feel angry and ruminate if you did not in fact help all your clients get better, but rather perhaps feel frustrated with yourself and then problem-solve other ways of helping them? (Criterion 2)
Example Response to Beginner Client Statement 2
How about something like, "If I get rejected, it only proves that I am human and maybe have some less-than-ideal traits or behaviors, but I am not a totally inadequate person"? (Criterion 1) Do you see how if you truly believed this, you certainly wouldn't feel happy, but probably something more like disappointment or sadness if you got rejected, and you would be less likely to isolate yourself? (Criterion 2)
Example Response to Beginner Client Statement 3
If you don't want to continue to feel guilty and avoid your friend, I propose you start thinking something such as, "I really wish I didn't lie to my friend, but there's nothing that says I absolutely must not." (Criterion 1) Do you understand that by truly believing this new idea, it will help you move from guilt to regret for lying to your friend, and will help you reach out rather than avoid your friend? (Criterion 2)
Example Response to Beginner Client Statement 4
To not feel anxious and get to that meeting, I would suggest something like, "Being disapproved of is really bad, but it is not the end of the world." (Criterion 1) Can you see that by believing this healthier way of thinking, you probably would feel that concern we discussed and do your best at the meeting? (Criterion 2)
Example Response to Beginner Client Statement 5
How about working on the following new belief: "I very much want him to pay more attention to me, but there is no reason he must do what I want"? (Criterion 1) Do you understand that thinking this way when he speaks to her will not result in your feeling nothing, but you might feel more sadness than jealousy? This could help you refrain from checking his phone, which is only making matters worse. (Criterion 2)

EXAMPLE RESPONSES TO INTERMEDIATE-LEVEL CLIENT STATEMENTS FOR EXERCISE 11

Example Response to Intermediate Client Statement 1

Would the following beliefs be helpful to you? "I really wish I had gotten that raise, but there's nothing that says I absolutely must have gotten it. My boss's decision to overlook me is a bad one, but a bad decision does not make him a total jerk as a person who can be helpful to you." (Criterion 1) Do you see how these rational beliefs could help you to feel frustrated or healthy anger toward your boss, which is your goal, and help you to accept him as a flawed person but not globally rate him? This new way of thinking could perhaps help you get a raise in the future. (Criterion 2)

Example Response to Intermediate Client Statement 2

I see you understand the connection between your irrational beliefs and your unhealthy depression and avoidance. What if you believed "I really want to have more social plans, but there is no absolute law of the universe that says I must. If I don't have more plans, all it says is that I failed at this goal at this particular time, but I am not a total failure as a person"? (Criterion 1) Can you see how believing this new idea will lead you to feel the sadness about your current situation rather than depression, and you would be more likely to approach people rather than avoid them? (Criterion 2)

Example Response to Intermediate Client Statement 3

What about thinking, "I wish I called my mother more, but there's no reason I absolutely must do so. If I don't, that choice may be bad, but that one choice does not define me as a totally bad person"? (Criterion 1) Can you see how believing this will change that guilt to regret or remorse and you would probably be more likely to pick up the phone when she calls you? (Criterion 2)

Example Response to Intermediate Client Statement 4

Would some helpful alternative beliefs be something like "I really don't want to make a mistake during my presentation, but I might and there's no reason I absolutely must not. If I do make a mistake, that would be really bad, but it would not be terrible"? (Criterion 1) If you believed these healthier, rational alternatives, would you feel healthier concern and not overprepare, which you stated were your goals? (Criterion 2)

Example Response to Intermediate Client Statement 5

Maybe a more helpful thought to change your jealousy would be "I wish my boyfriend showed me love, but there is no law that says he must do what I want. If he doesn't show me love, his behavior does not define my worth as a person." (Criterion 1) Can you see how these new beliefs will make you feel more disappointed than jealous when he doesn't show you love, and you will be less likely to nag him and possibly make your relationship decline? (Criterion 2)

EXAMPLE RESPONSES TO ADVANCED-LEVEL CLIENT STATEMENTS FOR EXERCISE 11

Example Response to Advanced Client Statement 1

What about thinking something like "I really want people to respect me, but there is no law that says they must do what I want. If they don't show me respect, I would dislike it, but I certainly could tolerate it. Not respecting me is a bad behavior, but that bad behavior does not make them totally incompetent morons"? (Criterion 1) If you really believed these new ideas, do you see how your goal of feeling frustrated and not being argumentative would be more likely achieved? (Criterion 2)

Example Response to Advanced Client Statement 2

How about thinking, "I really, really wish I didn't have so much loss in my life but unfortunately, there is nothing that says I must not have it. It's incredibly difficult to experience, but I can bear it. My situation is very bad, but it's not awful or the end of the world"? (Criterion 1) Can you see that strengthening your conviction in these new beliefs will help you move toward sadness and not spend so much time ruminating about your loss, which is what your goals are? (Criterion 2)

Example Response to Advanced Client Statement 3

What if I propose the following different, healthier beliefs: "I wish I had gone to my parents' anniversary party but there's no reason I absolutely should have. Not going was a bad decision, but that one bad decision does not totally define me as a bad person. The thought of facing them is difficult for me, but I can certainly stand it"? (Criterion 1) If you truly believed this new way of thinking, do you think that you would be more likely to achieve your goals of feeling remorse about your decision and call them? (Criterion 2)

Example Response to Advanced Client Statement 4

My suggestion is the following for healthier beliefs: "I strongly prefer making a good impression with my coworkers, but there is no absolute law that says I must. If I don't make a good impression, I would dislike that, but I would tolerate it. If I don't make a good impression, all that says is that I failed at this task, but that does not define me as a total failure as a person." (Criterion 1) Do you understand that believing these new ideas strongly in your gut will help you to achieve your goal of being concerned about the impression you leave and will probably help you not to act "weird" around them? (Criterion 2)

Example Response to Advanced Client Statement 5

I would propose the following healthier alternatives to your current beliefs: "I wish he would shower me with attention and love, but there's no law that says I must get what I want. If he doesn't do this, it would be really unpleasant and bad, but not awful. His lack of attention and love toward me does not define me as a worthless person." (Criterion 1) Do you understand that if you really believed these new rational alternatives, it would help you feel sadness about his behavior toward you and will also help you not to be so needy around him? (Criterion 2)

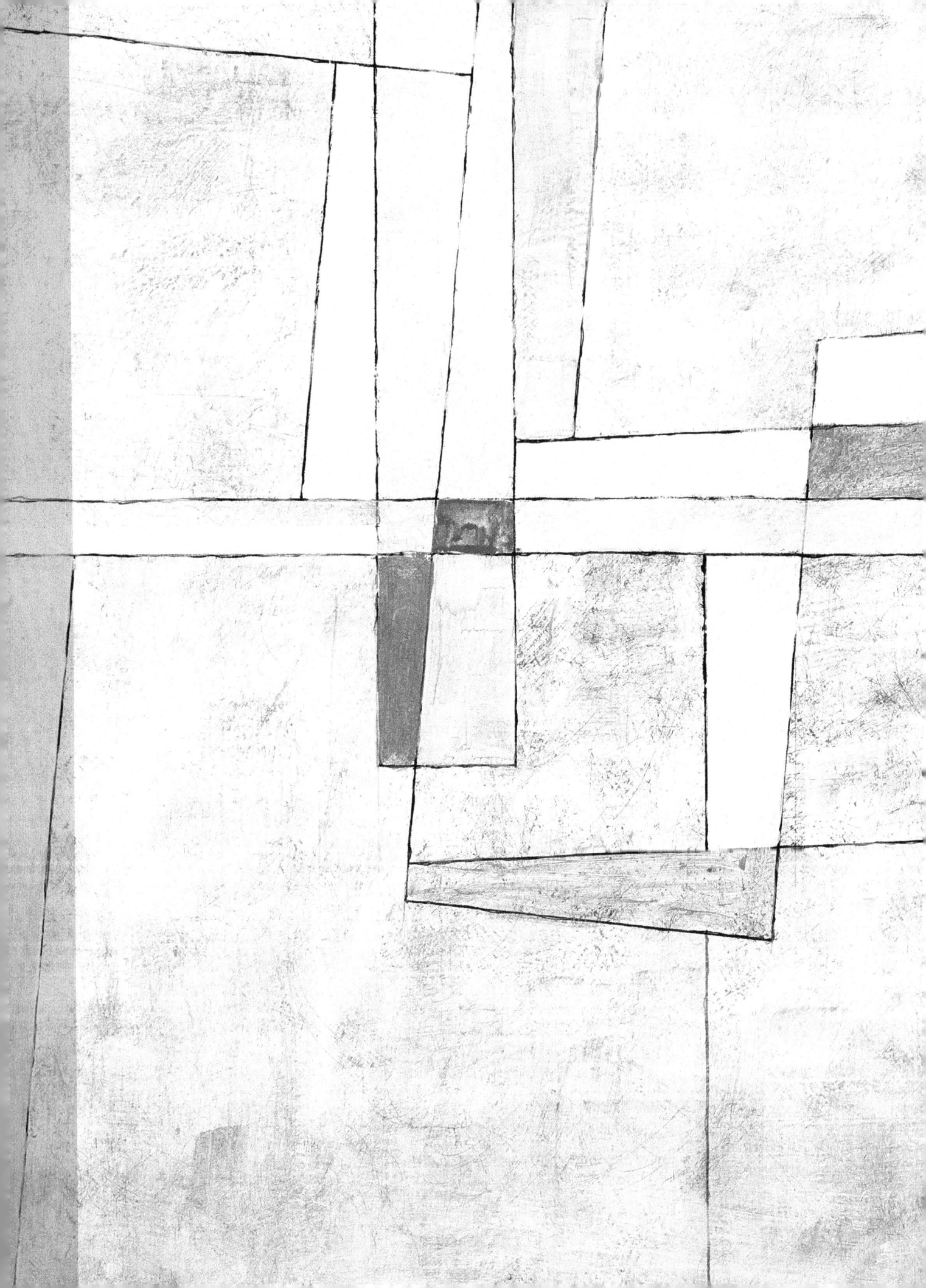

Collaborative Homework Development

Preparations for Exercise 12

1. Read the instructions in Chapter 2.

2. Download the Deliberate Practice Reaction Form and the Deliberate Practice Diary Form at https://www.apa.org/pubs/books/deliberate-practice-rational-emotive-behavior-therapy (see the "Clinician and Practitioner Resources" tab; also available in Appendixes A and B, respectively).

Skill Description

Skill Difficulty Level: Advanced

At the onset of the development of the theory and practice of rational emotive behavior therapy (REBT), Albert Ellis (1957, 1962) stressed the importance of homework assignments in between sessions to allow clients the opportunity to practice a healthier way of thinking, feeling, and behaving. Although assignment of behavioral homework is more measurable and easier to establish, having clients practice cognitive change might further increase the likelihood of their completion of behavioral assignments. This is the last skill listed among the exercises, but the development of homework is consistent throughout the practice of REBT regardless of the stage of therapy. Homework is negotiated and expected at each point of therapy to reinforce skills learned to promote clients' progress toward healthier ways of thinking, feeling, and behaving. Tailoring the homework to the client, providing a rationale for why doing the homework would be important for the client, and working to uncover any obstacles that might prevent homework from being done are all important components of homework in REBT.

Beginning homework assignments typically focus on teaching clients how to identify their activating events and unhealthy negative emotions, followed by assignments

https://doi.org/10.1037/0000334-014

Deliberate Practice in Rational Emotive Behavior Therapy, by M. D. Terjesen, K. A. Doyle, R. A. DiGiuseppe, A. Vaz, and T. Rousmaniere

to identify their irrational beliefs and understand the role of irrational beliefs in the development and maintenance of their unhealthy emotions and maladaptive behaviors. Intermediate homework assignments might involve having clients write out and dispute their irrational beliefs before and while they are experiencing unhealthy negative emotions. Later homework assignments often involve negotiating with clients to engage in behaviors that reinforce their exposure to feared stimuli, or engagement in adaptive behaviors such behaving assertively or engaging in mastery activities. For example, having clients engage in exposure behaviors that they previously believed would be "too difficult to handle" or that if they did the assignment, it would be "awful," overcomes their fears and strengthens the healthier rational beliefs that "it might be difficult, but I can handle this" and "it's bad but not awful" to do this. We recommend consulting DiGiuseppe et al. (2014) and Dryden (2001), who outline a variety of cognitive, emotional, and behavioral homework assignments. Cognitive homework assignments might include reading self-help books on REBT that review the philosophy of the therapy. Emotional homework assignments might include imagining occurrence of the activating event followed by images of experiencing the new healthy, adaptive negative emotions. Behavioral homework assignments might include exposure to feared stimuli, behaving assertively, or behavioral activation.

Finally, REBT practitioners work collaboratively with clients to develop the homework assignments. Doing this will help reinforce the rationale behind the specific homework assignment while also demonstrating to the client that they have therapeutic responsibility, which includes homework assignments. We have found that working collaboratively strengthens clients' commitment to completing homework, which has been linked to clinical outcomes. It has also been demonstrated that having the client identify specific times that they will do the work increases their compliance.

Special Considerations for Performing This Exercise

Each of the three levels of client statement reflects a different point in therapy so clinicians can practice collaborative development of homework assignments at the various stages of REBT. The homework assignments for the beginner-level statements should focus on having clients demonstrate and practice their understanding of the ABC model. The assignments for the intermediate-level statements should focus on disputing irrational beliefs. The assignments for the advanced statements should involve both behavior and cognitive change strategies.

SKILL CRITERIA FOR EXERCISE 12
1. The clinician proposes a homework assignment with the client that is aligned with clinical goals.
2. The clinician asks the client to set a specific day, time, and place to complete the homework.
3. The clinician assesses the presence of any practical, emotional, or cognitive obstacles that would make homework completion more challenging and less likely.

Examples of Collaborative Homework Development

Example 1

CLIENT: [*angry*] You are saying that technically she doesn't make me angry and that I am ultimately in control of my emotions, but now what?

THERAPIST: That is a fair question. Perhaps we could help you feel a healthier emotion. We could develop some between-session assignments that help you understand the relationship between beliefs, feelings, and behavior. You might write down or record on your phone when you get angry this week, and for each anger episode, you could record the situation and your thoughts and note what you did or did not do behaviorally. (Criterion 1) It may be helpful to set a certain time of day to practice and review these thoughts. (Criterion 2) Is there anything that you that could occur this week that would stop you from doing this homework? (Criterion 3)

Example 2

CLIENT: [*anxious*] Whenever I sit down to get work done, I get so anxious and overwhelmed. I start those "what if" thoughts we talked about, like "What if I won't get it all done?" I definitely do some catastrophizing at this point.

THERAPIST: I think it's terrific that you can identify that when you feel anxious and avoid doing the work that you are engaging in some awfulizing or catastrophizing. To help work toward the goal of feeling concerned about getting the work done rather than anxious, how about you challenge those catastrophizing beliefs? As you said, those beliefs occur when you sit down to do work. This might be a good opportunity to have you write down some disputes or challenges of these beliefs. (Criterion 1) Perhaps setting a specific time to review these thoughts and practice challenging them would be good. (Criterion 2) Is there anything that would get in your way of completing this task? (Criterion 3)

Example 3

CLIENT: [*depressed*] Losing my husband at this point in my life really was difficult. I used to have a lot of friends, but I don't have much of a social circle now, and the idea of reaching out or trying to make new friends seems frightening. Despite our work together, it still seems too difficult to do.

THERAPIST: Yes, losing him was tough and certainly contributes to your depression. We agreed that the goal of having social support to help you is a good one, but some of your beliefs about losing him interfere with your pursuit of new friends. This might be a good opportunity for you to practice the healthier belief of "It's difficult, but not too difficult" and then reach out to people this week. (Criterion 1) Maybe we can discuss specifics as to how many people you will reach out to this week. (Criterion 2) Besides those beliefs about it being "too difficult" that we know how to challenge, is there anything else that you think would stop you from doing it this week? (Criterion 3)

INSTRUCTIONS FOR EXERCISE 12

Step 1: Role-Play and Feedback

- The client says the first beginner client statement. The therapist **improvises** a response based on the skill criteria.
- The trainer (or if not available, the client) provides **brief** feedback based on the skill criteria.
- The client then repeats the same statement, and the therapist again improvises a response. The trainer (or client) again provides brief feedback.

Step 2: Repeat

- Repeat Step 1 for all the statements **in the current difficulty level** (beginner, intermediate, or advanced).

Step 3: Assess and Adjust Difficulty

- The therapist completes the Deliberate Practice Reaction Form (see Appendix A) and decides whether to make the exercise easier or harder or to repeat the same difficulty level.

Step 4: Repeat for Approximately 15 Minutes

- Repeat Steps 1 to 3 for at least 15 minutes.
- The trainees then switch therapist and client roles and start over.

Now it's your turn! Follow Steps 1 and 2 from the instructions.

Remember: The goal of the role-play is for trainees to practice improvising responses to the client statements in a manner that (a) uses the skill criteria and (b) feels authentic for the trainee. **Example therapist responses for each client statement are provided at the end of this exercise. Trainees should attempt to improvise their own responses before reading the example responses.**

BEGINNER-LEVEL CLIENT STATEMENTS FOR EXERCISE 12
Beginner Client Statement 1
[Angry] I understand that thinking she shouldn't act this way when she does doesn't help me. But what do I do in the moment when I get so worked up and angry?
Beginner Client Statement 2
[Depressed] Nothing is easy, even challenging these beliefs that make me depressed.
Beginner Client Statement 3
[Guilty] I really don't like feeling this way and recognize that even if she says things that aren't nice, that I am the one who ultimately decides just how guilty I feel. But what do I do when these overwhelming feelings of guilt occur?
Beginner Client Statement 4
[Anxious] I have done better with sleep hygiene and have gone to bed earlier and reduced my caffeine intake and technology exposure before going to bed, but these "what if" thoughts keep occurring at night that really stop me from sleeping or at the very least I know it will be a bad night's sleep. What can I do about these thoughts?
Beginner Client Statement 5
[Jealous] My partner at work gets this praise heaped upon her—more than she deserves. Our whole team is attending an event where she is getting recognized again. I want to be there to support her, but the jealousy I experience will probably be my plus-one to the event and make me quite miserable at it. I want to go, but should I?

Assess and adjust the difficulty before moving to the next difficulty level (see Step 3 in the exercise instructions).

INTERMEDIATE-LEVEL CLIENT STATEMENTS FOR EXERCISE 12
Intermediate Client Statement 1
[Angry] I understand that I have those demanding beliefs when I get angry. But I am still thinking they are true. I have a hard time changing them.
Intermediate Client Statement 2
[Depressed] When I question the beliefs, I see they are ridiculous. But a part of me still thinks they are true. How do I change those thoughts?
Intermediate Client Statement 3
[Guilty] I see how these beliefs make me feel guilty. But I have a hard time not condemning myself for what I did wrong. How do I stop condemning myself?
Intermediate Client Statement 4
[Anxious] Those "what if" thoughts keep popping into my head. If those bad things did happen, I believe it would be just awful. How do I stop thinking that those events would be so terrible?
Intermediate Client Statement 5
[Jealous] If I go to the event honoring my sister, I can probably stand it, but I will still feel jealous and think that I deserve some recognition. How do I go about not having these jealous thoughts?

 Assess and adjust the difficulty before moving to the next difficulty level (see Step 3 in the exercise instructions).

ADVANCED-LEVEL CLIENT STATEMENTS FOR EXERCISE 12
Advanced Client Statement 1
[Angry] I see from what we talk about that my anger toward my landlord is only hurting me and not changing him. But I still think that I'm right and he should give me a partial rent reduction for not having heat in the building during the coldest week of the year. Not sure what my next step is here.
Advanced Client Statement 2
[Depressed] I really believe it will be too hard to get myself out of the apartment and take a walk, even though I know it will make me feel better. How do I get myself to do something I know is good for me, when I haven't been able to do so yet?
Advanced Client Statement 3
[Guilty] I see how I'm being hypocritical when I give others a "pass" if they screw up and I condemn myself when I do. But I just can't seem to let go of my rules of how I should act and what it means about me when I break those rules. How do I get beyond this and be kinder to myself? I don't want to continue walking around with all this guilt.
Advanced Client Statement 4
[Anxious] I'm sorry, but even though we've gone over this repeatedly, I still think that my anxiety helps me to do well in school. Not sure what to do about my anxiety. I believe that if I replace my anxiety with concern about my school performance, everything is going to fall to pieces.
Advanced Client Statement 5
[Jealous] I know my jealousy is only adding more problems to my relationship. I can see how feeling disappointed or even sad about my partner's lack of attention to me would be more helpful. I just am not sure how I can get to that other place. Where do I start?

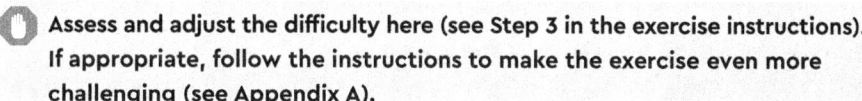 **Assess and adjust the difficulty here** (see Step 3 in the exercise instructions). If appropriate, follow the instructions to make the exercise even more challenging (see Appendix A).

Example Therapist Responses: Collaborative Homework Development

Remember: Trainees should attempt to improvise their own responses before reading the example responses. **Do not read the following responses verbatim unless you are having trouble coming up with your own responses!**

EXAMPLE RESPONSES TO BEGINNER-LEVEL CLIENT STATEMENTS FOR EXERCISE 12
Example Response to Beginner Client Statement 1
I think it's great that you recognize that those thoughts don't help you to manage your anger. It might be helpful to know when you are most upset or angry, what those beliefs are, how long the feeling lasts for, and any behaviors that go along with it. Perhaps as homework you can write up what happened, what were you thinking, how you felt, and what you did. (Criterion 1) Perhaps start by looking for the week ahead and finding time to plan for situations that you may get angry in and set up a system to write down these thoughts in advance. (Criterion 2) Do you think there is anything that may occur this week that would stop you from doing this homework? (Criterion 3)
Example Response to Beginner Client Statement 2
Challenging these beliefs can be difficult and requires an awareness of the beliefs that led to the depression to begin with. Like most things, this awareness will become easier with practice. If we wait until the moment that we feel depressed, it may be even more difficult. To start, let's discuss how to get you to assess these beliefs and the situations that they are most likely to occur in. Perhaps writing these beliefs down when you find yourself feeling depressed would be a good start. (Criterion 1) Maybe initially write down and challenge these beliefs three times a day before each meal. (Criterion 2) Would there be anything you think that would stop you from doing this? (Criterion 3)
Example Response to Beginner Client Statement 3
Good recognition that you are in control of your emotional experience. You can probably predict with a good deal of accuracy that she will continue to say things that are not nice. Maybe you can write down or record those helpful beliefs and, before interacting with her, remind yourself of those helpful beliefs that we generated to make you feel regret instead of guilt. (Criterion 1) Looking at your calendar and planning for an interaction with her and reviewing helpful thoughts that lead to helpful emotions and behaviors before you meet with her would be a good start. (Criterion 2) You cannot control what she will do, but is there anything that you believe may stop you from doing this homework and build up some immunity to the guilt? (Criterion 3)
Example Response to Beginner Client Statement 4
Great that you have done the previous homework on healthy sleep hygiene. You also pointed out some unhealthy "what if" thoughts. Before we develop several challenges of these thoughts, it may be helpful to look at what are the specific "what if" thoughts you have and when you have them during the night. Let's predict you will have these beliefs nightly and have you write down what they are. (Criterion 1) While you can probably predict what these thoughts will be, maybe keep a pad by your bedside and jot them down when you have them. (Criterion 2) You have done great at integrating the other exercises into your nightly routine. Is there anything you can think of that would interfere with your ability to implement this as well? (Criterion 3)

Example Response to Beginner Client Statement 5

If you want to go and support her, it would be helpful to be aware of what the beliefs are that lead to you feeling jealous. (Criterion 1) The event is in 2 weeks, and you have been to similar events in the past. Maybe you can spend 10 to 15 minutes a night where you can imagine the situation and others recognizing her and then you try and become aware of those beliefs that lead you to feel jealous. (Criterion 2) What are your thoughts about this? Do you think it will be helpful, and is there anything that may stop you from using this strategy? (Criterion 3)

EXAMPLE RESPONSES TO INTERMEDIATE-LEVEL CLIENT STATEMENTS FOR EXERCISE 12

Example Response to Intermediate Client Statement 1

OK, let's discuss some things you could do between session to help you change your anger at her; perhaps you can fill out these ABC homework sheets and challenge the beliefs that occur with your anger. (Criterion 1) Maybe you could do an ABC sheet once a day? (Criterion 2) Can you think of anything that would stop you from doing this assignment? (Criterion 3)

Example Response to Intermediate Client Statement 2

So we want to identify a task that will help you change your depression, such as writing down disputes of the beliefs related to your depression. (Criterion 1) Is there a time of day you can agree to do that? (Criterion 2) Are there any events, thoughts, or emotions that would stop you from doing this? (Criterion 3)

Example Response to Intermediate Client Statement 3

It would be good to come up with some activities that will help you change your guilt to remorse. Could you spend some time each day imagining what you did wrong and focus on the new emotion of remorse? (Criterion 1) Now think of a good time for you to do this imagery each day. (Criterion 2) Can you think of anything or any thoughts or emotions that would stop you from completing this assignment? (Criterion 3)

Example Response to Intermediate Client Statement 4

It is good you recognize the role those thoughts play in your emotions. And we want to come up with some things that you can do to challenge the awfulizing you do. Perhaps you can spend some time writing down challenges to the idea that the "what if" events are awful. (Criterion 1) You could pick a time each day to do such a task. (Criterion 2) Can you think of anything that would stop you from practicing this activity? (Criterion 3)

Example Response to Intermediate Client Statement 5

I think it would be helpful to have you practice some activity that will get you to give up the demand that you should get recognition too. Perhaps you can imagine being at your sister's award ceremony and imagine thinking, "I want recognition, but I don't have to have it now. This is her day." (Criterion 1) Can you identify a specific time each day you could do this for five minutes? (Criterion 2) Now, can you think of anything, a thought or an emotion, that would stop you from doing this? (Criterion 3)

EXAMPLE RESPONSES TO ADVANCED-LEVEL CLIENT STATEMENTS FOR EXERCISE 12

Example Response to Advanced Client Statement 1

You've been very clear about identifying all the ways in which your anger is only having a negative impact on you. You may be right that your landlord should give you a rent reduction, but the reality is that he is not going to. If you really believed in your gut the alternative belief "I really wish my landlord would act differently, but there is no reason that says he must," will it help you replace that unhealthy anger with healthier, strong annoyance? Rehearsal of these healthier beliefs is important. (Criterion 1) It may be helpful to rehearse that healthier, rational belief at times during the day when you are not activated, such as on your way to work or while you're in the shower. (Criterion 2) Is there anything that you can think of, either emotionally or practically, that would get in the way of you doing this exercise? (Criterion 3)

Example Response to Advanced Client Statement 2

It sounds like your irrational belief that taking a walk would be too hard is what will stop you from doing what will help you get out of this depression. For this week's homework, perhaps to prepare for taking the walk, you might consider putting together a closing argument as if you were an attorney in front of a judge and jury persuading them as to why it will be hard, but not too hard, and rehearse it over and over with force. That way, you will begin convincing yourself of that same idea. (Criterion 1) Let's figure out the best date and time and how often you want to commit to doing this. (Criterion 2) Can you identify anything this week that might prevent you from doing this homework assignment? (Criterion 3)

Example Response to Advanced Client Statement 3

You are clear you don't want to feel this guilt you've been walking around with when you don't do as you believe you should and continue thinking you're a horrible person. I think a good homework assignment would be for you to keep practice challenging these unhealthy beliefs. (Criterion 1) Perhaps spending a specific time each day challenging those two irrational beliefs from a functional, empirical, and logical perspective would be helpful, even writing down your disputes against these beliefs. (Criterion 2) Is there anything that you can predict before we end the session that could get in the way of you doing this assignment? (Criterion 3)

Example Response to Advanced Client Statement 4

I hear the hesitation you have about changing your anxiety to concern regarding your school performance. In REBT, we often suggest clients consider a hedonic calculus, or a cost–benefit analysis of the short- and long-term advantages and disadvantages of keeping your anxiety. You may want to evaluate whether this anxiety is working for you. (Criterion 1) Let's discuss what would be the best time for you to commit to making this list. (Criterion 2) Can you think of anything that might get in the way of you completing this before our next session that we should troubleshoot? (Criterion 3)

Example Response to Advanced Client Statement 5

As you said, your jealousy is only getting in the way of your relationship. So, there is a dysfunctionality that the beliefs that lead to that emotion block you from working toward your goal. Focusing on this functional dispute of your beliefs as they relate to your goal of feeling disappointed or sad about your relationship may be a helpful between-session assignment. (Criterion 1) It may be helpful if you spent several times a day over the next week doing this. (Criterion 2) Can you come up with any roadblocks that would get in the way of doing this—such as time constraints, forgetting, or not feeling like doing it—that we should address before the session ends? (Criterion 3)

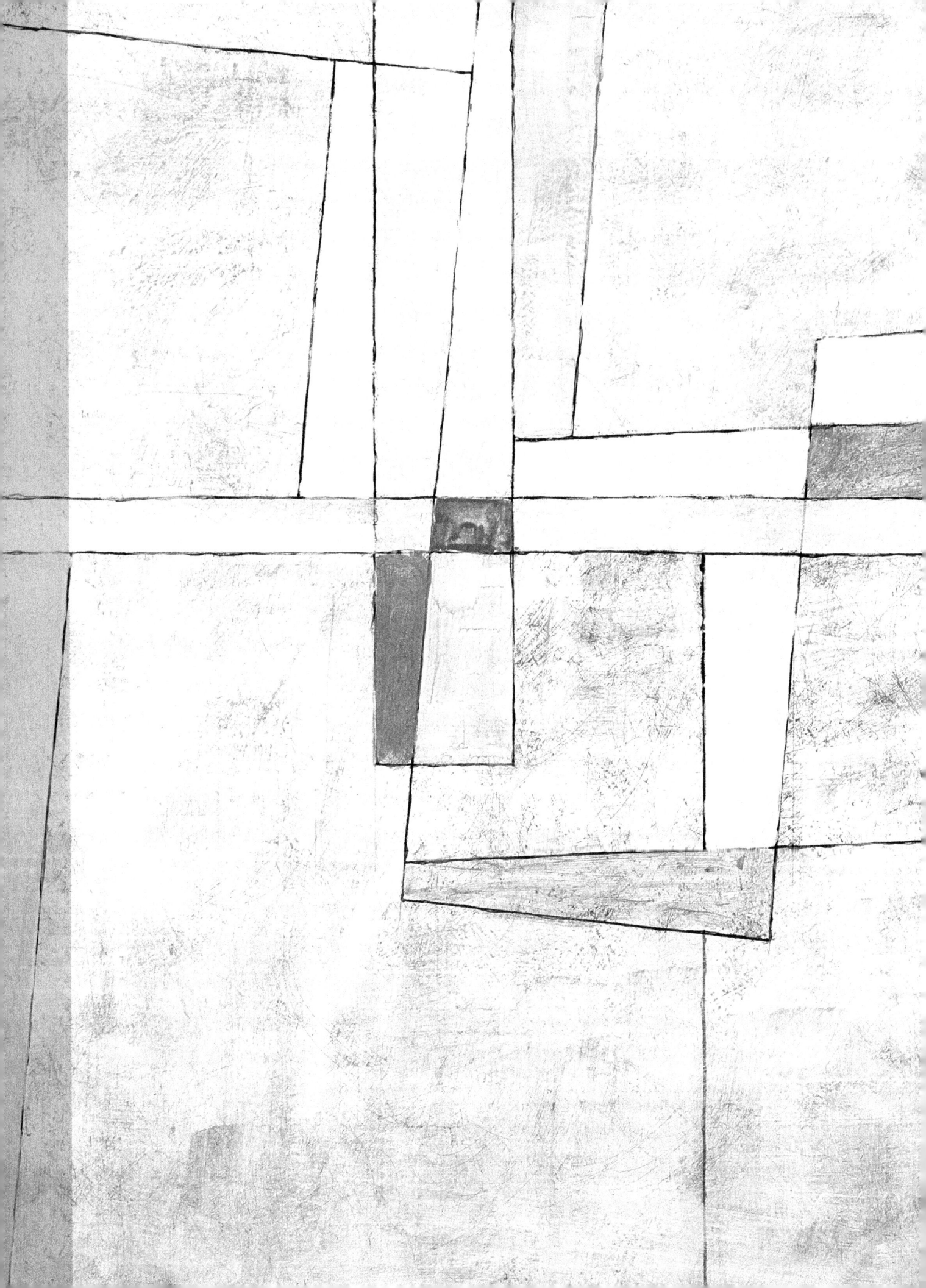

Annotated Rational Emotive Behavior Therapy Practice Session Transcript

It is now time to put all the skills you have learned together! This exercise presents a transcript from a typical rational emotive behavior therapy (REBT) session. Each therapist statement is annotated to indicate which REBT skill from Exercises 1 through 12 is used. This transcript provides an example of how therapists can interweave many different REBT skills in response to clients.

Instructions

As in the previous exercises, one trainee can play the client while the other plays the therapist. As much as possible, the trainee who plays the client should try to adopt an authentic, emotional tone as if they were a real client. The first time through, both partners can read verbatim from the transcript. After one complete run-through, try it again. This time, the client can read from the script while the therapist can improvise to the degree that they feel comfortable. At this point, you may also want to reflect on it with a supervisor and go through it again. Before you start, it is recommended that both therapist and client read the entire transcript through on your own, until the end. The purpose of the sample transcript is to give trainees the opportunity to try out what it is like to offer the REBT responses in a sequence that mimics live therapy sessions.

Note to Therapists

Remember to be aware of your vocal quality. Match your tone to the client's presentation. Thus, if the clients present vulnerable, soft emotions behind their words, soften your tone to be soothing and calm. If clients on the other hand, are aggressive and angry, match your tone to be firm.

https://doi.org/10.1037/0000334-015

Deliberate Practice in Rational Emotive Behavior Therapy, by M. D. Terjesen, K. A. Doyle, R. A. DiGiuseppe, A. Vaz, and T. Rousmaniere

Annotated REBT Transcript

THERAPIST 1: Hi, [client's name], it's nice to meet you.

CLIENT 1: Nice to meet you as well.

THERAPIST 2: So, I realize that this type of therapy, rational emotive behavior therapy, or more commonly referred to as REBT, is new to you. I'm wondering if before we get started, is it OK if I explain a little bit more about what REBT is? You had mentioned that someone recommended you try REBT, but in our initial phone discussion, you indicated that you were unfamiliar with it.

CLIENT 2: Yes, I would love to understand more about it and how and if you think this approach can help me.

THERAPIST 3: Great. Many people who come in for therapy have this idea that somebody or something or some situation is what's causing them or making them feel a certain way, like angry, anxious, depressed or hurt, or act in a certain way, like getting really verbally aggressive. People will say things like "because this person does this, I need a drink," or "I'm so depressed I need to go online and do some shopping," or "He makes me so anxious!" So, they have this idea that these outside events, situations, or people are what is creating their problems emotionally and behaviorally. In REBT, we refer to these outside events or situations as the activating event, or "A." In REBT, we don't discount the fact that those outside events are a part of what contributes to our emotional or behavioral disturbance. However, we focus more on the way you look at what's happening, or your beliefs, the "Bs," about the activating event, that cause those emotional and behavioral upsets, referred to as consequences, or "Cs." Those emotional and behavioral responses can be either healthy and adaptive or unhealthy and maladaptive, depending on the beliefs you're holding about the activating event. The same situation can occur to two different people, and they can have two very different reactions emotionally and behaviorally because they're thinking differently about what that situation means to them. Does that make sense? Do you have any questions or doubts about this ABC model? (Skill 1: Psychoeducation About REBT's ABC Model)

CLIENT 3: So basically, you're telling me that my sister is not the cause of my anger?

THERAPIST 4: Unfortunately, I am. I'm not discounting that she is an activating event for you, but you'll see when we take an example that your anger is largely coming from what you're thinking about or telling yourself about her or her actions that's creating your anger. The bad news is that we may not be able to change your sister, but the good news is that if she doesn't change, we can change the way you think about your sister to help you with your reactions.

CLIENT 4: I got it. That makes sense. But I still would like her to change . . .

THERAPIST 5: I know, believe me I know. I have a sister too! But we're better off starting to change what we can, which is our thinking. Let's go back to what I mentioned a few minutes ago about your emotional and behavioral reactions to an activating event. Assuming the activating event is negative, which your sister's behavior may be, we can respond with emotions and behaviors that are considered healthy negative emotions (HNEs) and adaptive behaviors or unhealthy negative emotions (UNEs) and maladaptive or dysfunctional behaviors. It's not realistic to think you are going to have a neutral reaction to a negative event. We're not looking to eliminate emotions. The important distinction we make in REBT is between unhealthy and healthy emotions and adaptive and maladaptive behaviors. If someone is experiencing a UNE, such as anxiety about giving a talk, they are often more likely to fumble on their words because they're anxious. If they were to be concerned about their talk, they probably would be more focused and less likely to fumble. So, you see, the UNEs get in the way of your goal achievement, whereas the HNEs are still negative but do not block goal attainment. In REBT, we propose that UNEs and maladaptive behaviors result from what we call irrational beliefs, which are very dogmatic, rigid beliefs that are illogical and block us from achieving our goals. HNEs and adaptive behaviors come from rational beliefs which are more flexible ideas that are logical and consistent with reality, and lead to goal attainment and better problem solving. I know this is a lot. Do you have any questions so far? (Skill 2: Psychoeducation About Dysfunctional Versus Functional Negative Emotions and Behaviors)

CLIENT 5: I don't think so. It's making sense, I think.

THERAPIST 6: Great. At any point stop me if you have a question. So, the last part that is important is that in REBT, we are not going to focus on reducing the intensity of your emotion. In other words, we're not going to help you to feel less anxious or less angry. That would be progress, but you would still be holding some irrational beliefs. Instead, we are going to work on you replacing your UNE with an HNE. So, replacing anxiety with concern, or depression with sadness, or guilt with remorse or regret. That way, we're changing your irrational thinking to a more rational philosophy and as a result changing your UNE to HNE as well as changing your negative behavioral responses to more healthy behavioral ones. Do you have any questions about that idea? (Skill 2: Psychoeducation About Dysfunctional Versus Functional Negative Emotions and Behaviors)

CLIENT 6: Not yet. I think it will get clearer as we talk about the situation with my sister.

THERAPIST 7: I agree. I think it would be helpful if we focus in on a specific problem that you're having, or that brought you in today. Is there a specific problem that you would like to discuss?

CLIENT 7: Yes, so my sister and I tend to butt heads more than we don't. I usually can keep myself together and feel annoyed, but there's those times when I tend to get angry at her and blow up about whatever's being said or done. She gets under my skin, and then I get very, very angry with her.

THERAPIST 8: Before we go further, you said that you usually can keep yourself together and feel annoyed, but there's those occasions where it escalates to anger. What's the difference for you when you're annoyed as opposed to angry?

CLIENT 8: My sister and I are complete opposites, like oil and water. I know we're not always going to get along or agree on things. And you know, in general, when people don't agree, sometimes it can get a little frustrating and you butt heads. But it's when it's constant. It's as if it's one thing after another and then another. My personality is usually to brush things under the rug, and then all of a sudden, that rug turns the little molehill into a mountain. And that's when I let it blow up.

THERAPIST 9: So just to throw it back to you to make sure that I'm understanding, what you do when you're annoyed is that you brush it under the rug, you kind of push through it, but eventually it gets to a boiling point, and then it erupts. Correct? And do you erupt?

CLIENT 9: I do. Sometimes it's calm and I'm like, "OK, you need to take a deep breath and leave because you're going to say something you regret."

THERAPIST 10: Is that when you're annoyed? Or is that when you're angry?

CLIENT 10: That's when I'm annoyed.

THERAPIST 11: So, when you're annoyed you are able to walk away because you're going to say something you might regret so you're thinking about the consequences of your actions?

CLIENT 11: Yes, that's right.

THERAPIST 12: OK, so would it be accurate for me to say that if you were angry and didn't walk away, there's a high probability that you would say something out of anger that you might regret later on?

CLIENT 12: Oh, probably as it's coming out, I'd probably say something harsh, and my face would probably go red. And then shortly after I'd think, "Oh, no, what did I just say?"

THERAPIST 13: Okay, what would be your goal for today? I heard the problem. But what is it exactly you want to accomplish?

CLIENT 13: So, while I really want my sister to change, I think my goal would be to not let the anger get the best of me or not let the anger get in the way of my relationship. I know I'm not going to get along with my sister every day. I know that and I've annoyingly accepted that usually, but I—I think it's just to not let the anger be such a big part of our relationship.

THERAPIST 14: Do you think it would be helpful if we could work on helping you not get angry at your sister? And perhaps, stay at the level of being annoyed when you know, you're very different personalities? You're not going to be happy, you know, unicorns, sunshine, all of that. Right? But perhaps being annoyed, where you said, you do push it under the rug. (Skill 3: Agreement on the Session Goals) Maybe later we can talk about more helpful behavioral strategies when you're annoyed, because it sounds like pushing it under the rug is almost like putting out a fire, but then another fire's going to come up in the next room at some point. Does that make sense?

CLIENT 14: Yes.

THERAPIST 15: OK, so for now, you said your goal is to work on your anger toward your sister and thereby not blow up at her. If you can give me a recent example of when you got angry at your sister, something that pops out in your head that's either recent or very salient?

CLIENT 15: Oh, yeah. So, she lives not far from us. And she makes comments to me, even recently, we were just there for dinner the other night. I'm 33 years old and living with my parents, but she lives not far from us. And our parents take care of her as well. So, the only difference between she and I is her location. That's literally the only difference.

THERAPIST 16: And so, what happened the other night at dinner, what occurred where you got angry and blew up at her?

CLIENT 16: She made a comment, as she often does, about how I'm 33 years old and living at home and mom and dad pay for everything for me. I always have to have the last comment, so I screamed in front of her two young kids, "That's rich coming from someone who lives in a brand-new home paid for by mom and dad. You know, every little nail and screw, every door handle, is all paid for by our parents. So, there's no difference between the two of us. You know, we're in the same circumstances, except you have a different address. But you know, actually, I'm more independent than you are in terms of financials, and maybe even life circumstances."

THERAPIST 17: And when you said this, that is when you got angry—when she made that comment?

CLIENT 17: Yes. Yes.

THERAPIST 18: OK. And that's when you pointed out that there's the screws in the wall, the door handles that your parents paid for, correct?

CLIENT 18: Correct.

THERAPIST 19: You can put an emotional label to how you felt; in this case, it was anger in that moment, and then you exploded. So just to make sure we are on the same page, your goal is to work on replacing your anger toward your sister with annoyance and then change your behavioral reaction of blowing up verbally with walking away or staying calm? Because when you say those things to your sister, it's like toothpaste that you can't get back into the tube. Are you in agreement that those emotional and behavioral goals make sense? (Skill 3: Agreement on the Session Goals)

CLIENT 19: Yeah, that make's sense.

THERAPIST 20: I want you to go back to that dinner when your sister made the comment about your parents paying for everything for you and you became angry. What were you thinking as you became angry? As she's saying what sounds like a snarky comment. What was going through your mind about what she was saying to get you to that emotion of anger instead of annoyance? That sounds like it's unhealthy because then you ended up saying things that you regret saying. Try to go back to that specific moment.

CLIENT 20: What was I thinking at that moment?

THERAPIST 21: Yes, thoughts to make you angry about what she was saying?

CLIENT 21: I blew up at her. I told her off.

THERAPIST 22: It's interesting, when I'm asking you what you were thinking as you got angry, you tell me what you did, which is not uncommon. Let's go back to what you were thinking as you got angry. So far, we've got the pot calling the kettle black. It sounds like you're thinking, "You know, we're in the same circumstances, except you have a different address. But you know actually, I'm more independent than you are in terms of financials, and maybe even life circumstances." Those are all what we call inferences or conclusions that you're drawing from what she's saying, which could be true or could be false. And you know, we could test those inferences out. But those inferences in and of themselves are not necessarily going to lead to your anger. Perhaps you also had some other beliefs, which we call irrational beliefs, which are rigid and dogmatic, expectations or demands about someone's behavior or exaggerations of how bad something is, or self- or other-condemnation that you were telling yourself besides those inferences. Do you think you did? (Skill 4: Clarifying Inferences From Irrational Beliefs)

CLIENT 22: Yes, I think that is probably true. But nothing I said was wrong.

THERAPIST 23: Let's suppose your inferences are true—you and your sister are in the same circumstances, except you have a different address. But actually, you are more independent than she is in terms of finances, and maybe even life circumstances. What else do you think you might have been telling yourself about her pot calling your kettle black that's creating your anger?

CLIENT 23: What was I thinking when I got so angry? She's worse off than me. She shouldn't be saying that we're in the same situation because I pay for all of my other stuff except for rent. And I hate to admit it, but I also think she's kind of a failure because she has to rely on my parents. (Skill 5: Assessing Irrational Beliefs About the Activating Event)

THERAPIST 24: OK. So, we have two irrational beliefs here that you mentioned that you experience when you're angry. One is "She shouldn't be saying that because we're in the same situation because I pay for all of my other stuff except for rent" and "She's a failure because she has to rely on my parents." Which of those two irrational beliefs do you think is more problematic for you that we should target first? (Skill 6: Prioritizing Which Irrational Beliefs to Target for Change)

CLIENT 24: I think I want to start with what she shouldn't be saying.

THERAPIST 25: So, we start with "She shouldn't be saying that we're in the same situation because I pay for all of my other stuff except for rent?"

CLIENT 25: Yes, that one.

THERAPIST 26: OK, [client's name], so going back to that dinner when your sister made her comment, can you see how telling yourself, "She **shouldn't** be saying that we're in the same situation because I pay for all of my other stuff except for rent," but in fact she is not recognizing this, that's what's causing you to feel angry? Can you see that connection and the result of becoming angry and blowing up? If she **should** act a certain way and she did act that certain way, you probably wouldn't get angry. Does that make sense? (Skill 7: Teaching the Belief–Consequence Connection)

CLIENT 26: I get that. I don't like it, but I get it.

THERAPIST 27: All right. So now that you see that your demand about how your sister should act is leading to your anger and blowing up at her in front of her kids, and you have identified that reacting with annoyance would be better for you, we're going to work on challenging or disputing this expectation, or demand that you have. I'm going to ask you different questions about this demand you have about her behavior. Are you ready?

CLIENT 27: I think so.

THERAPIST 28: OK, [client's name], how does holding onto the belief "She shouldn't be saying that we're in the same situation because I pay for all of my stuff except for rent" help you to achieve your goal of being annoyed and not blowing up at her?

CLIENT 28: It doesn't help me at all. I just get angry and say things I regret.

THERAPIST 29: OK, so then tell me how this belief "She shouldn't be saying that we're in the same situation because I pay all of my other stuff except for rent" creates problems for you?

CLIENT 29: Like I said, I get angry. I say things I regret. I then ruminate about what she said, and it spills into the rest of my day. I get snippy with other people for no reason.

THERAPIST 30: So, what I'm hearing is that this demand about your sister's behavior is not working at all for you but seems to be causing even more problems for you because you have her annoying behavior that's not changing and now you have this anger and its consequences on your life. Is that correct? (Skill 8: Functional Disputation of Irrational Beliefs)

CLIENT 30: True.

THERAPIST 31: OK, let's look at this demand from a different angle. This might be a tough one, but remember, your goal is to work toward replacing that anger with annoyance. So, [client's name], where is it written that your sister **should** or **must** act the way you want her to? Which sibling relationship guidebook that has been written about how sisters, brothers, family, and people must act should I check out of the library? Please tell me so I can show it to my sister! [*laughs*]

CLIENT 31: Libraries don't carry this book. There's only one copy, and it's in my head. [*laughs*]

THERAPIST 32: Believe me, [client's name], I have a **lot** of things written in my head that only if they were true—like I **should** win the lottery! But that hasn't happened. So, is there some law I am not aware of that says your sister **should/must** do what you want? (Skill 9: Empirical Disputation of Irrational Beliefs)

CLIENT 32: [*sighs*] Unfortunately, no. I see your point.

THERAPIST 33: So, there's no law. There's no law that says that people have to act the way we want them to, even if it would lead to better consequences. Right? That's a tough pill to swallow. The alternative, which would be what's preferable regarding her behavior, would have such better outcomes, but we can't control her. What's your reaction to that?

CLIENT 33: Um, I mean, you're not wrong, it's certainly a tough pill to swallow. But I get it.

THERAPIST 34: Let's look at your demand from a different perspective. If we define "shoulds" as essentials or absolute "have-tos," does your "should" about your sister's behavior meet that criteria or definition of the word? Is she free to make bad choices and not always do the right thing like you are demanding? (Skill 10: Semantic Disputation of Irrational Beliefs)

CLIENT 34: Saying it that way, I guess not. It's not an absolute that she act a certain way. But it definitely would be so much better!

THERAPIST 35: I agree, it would be better if she acted differently, but it's not an absolute that she should or must. Let's summarize what we've gotten from these challenges or disputes of that demand so far. You see that your demand of your sister's behavior is not working for you, but rather it's actually working against you in terms of your goals of being annoyed and walking away or staying calm but rather you become angry and then verbally aggressive. This demand is not written anywhere except in your head. There's no evidence or law that says she **must** act according to how you want her to. And finally, your definition of "should" does not meet the criteria for absolutes. Did I sum it up correctly?

CLIENT 35: Yes, that about sums it up.

THERAPIST 36: It's great that you see your demand of your sister's behavior is problematic. We now need to come up with a new healthier idea or belief about her behavior, what we call rational alternatives, to replace your demanding irrational belief. An idea that has more flexibility to it, is consistent with reality, and won't keep creating that anger and verbal blowups. Can you think of anything that would help you to feel more annoyance when your sister acts that way rather than anger?

CLIENT 36: What about, "Here she goes again. I hate when she does this."

THERAPIST 37: That's good. And that hopefully will help you in that moment. What those statements are not going to do though is help change your demanding philosophy about your sister to something more flexible. We need a laser focus on your demand and negate it so you can't sneak back in a should. I explain this to clients by having them imagine an iron gate that is open, and the goal is to have it brought down to the ground, so no people or vehicles can get in under it. When we construct the rational alternative to our irrational belief, we need to make sure that gate is down to the ground. Do you have any questions so far? Does this make sense?

CLIENT 37: Yes, I think it makes sense, and I don't think I have any questions yet. Maybe I'll hear the rest of what you're saying, and I might have some then.

THERAPIST 38: Fair enough. There is a lot to digest here. OK, so let's restate your demand, and maybe condense it for now: "My sister shouldn't be saying that." The full rational alternative to this demand would be the following: "I wish (or really wish) my sister didn't say this, but there's no reason she should/must not." Can you see how the gate is now on the ground? Do you understand that if you really believed this new thought that you would be more likely to experience a healthy negative emotion like annoyance? (Skill 11: Constructing Full Rational Alternative Beliefs to Replace Irrational Beliefs)

CLIENT 38: Um, I think so.

THERAPIST 39: Well, let me try and help make this clearer. Let's say we said, "I wish (really wish) my sister didn't say this" and we left it there. At this point, the gate is half-closed. You can sneak back under the gate with "And she **shouldn't**!" We need to close the gate, and we do so by negating the irrational demand with "But there's no reason she should/ must not." Any questions about this?

CLIENT 39: No, I get it. That makes sense. I have to remember to close the gate . . .

THERAPIST 40: Or else?

CLIENT 40: My "should" will walk right through and I'll get angry and say or do something I would later regret.

THERAPIST 41: Excellent! How do you think you will feel if you really believe in your gut, through rehearsal, the new rational belief, "I wish my sister didn't say this, but there's no reason she should or must not"?

CLIENT 41: If I really believe this, I am not going to be happy, but I won't be angry. I think I will feel annoyed and then not blow up.

THERAPIST 42: Yes! OK, so, based on what we talked about today, is there anything you think would be helpful as a homework assignment? Something to practice, let's say? (Skill 12: Collaborative Homework Development)

CLIENT 42: I didn't love the disputing that we did because, you know, it made me realize that some of my thinking isn't working for me, so I think that's probably what I should focus on this week. Because if I didn't like it, it probably means it's important for me to replace my anger with annoyance toward my sister.

THERAPIST 43: I commend you on that insight and your high frustration tolerance of doing this exercise. So, specifically, what are you going to do?

CLIENT 43: I'm going to challenge my demand about my sister when she starts saying something that's offensive with the questions we went over today.

THERAPIST 44: Great! Can I make a suggestion?

CLIENT 44: Sure.

THERAPIST 45: How about we don't wait until your sister says something offensive to you to start challenging your demand? My concern is that it may be too late at that point because your default way of thinking—that demandingness—will most likely kick in, and you'll find yourself angry and do or say something you may regret. What do you think about practicing the disputes when you're not activated by her? Is there a time of day where you're alone and can focus on your demand and do the disputing exercise?

CLIENT 45: Uhhh, yeah. When I'm showering, no one is bothering me.

THERAPIST 46: Well, that's a relief. [*laughing*] Great. So, when you're showering, you're going to practice challenging the demand you have of your sister. I think it's good to think of this as it being like building a muscle. The more repetition you do, the stronger the muscle becomes.

CLIENT 46: Got it.

THERAPIST 47: Great. One more thing before I let you go. Can you anticipate anything that might get in the way of you doing this homework assignment? Any emotional or practical obstacles that would get in the way? (Skill 12: Collaborative Homework Development)

CLIENT 47: Besides not showering, I don't think so.

THERAPIST 48: Excellent. So, I will see you next week and we'll see how you did with the homework.

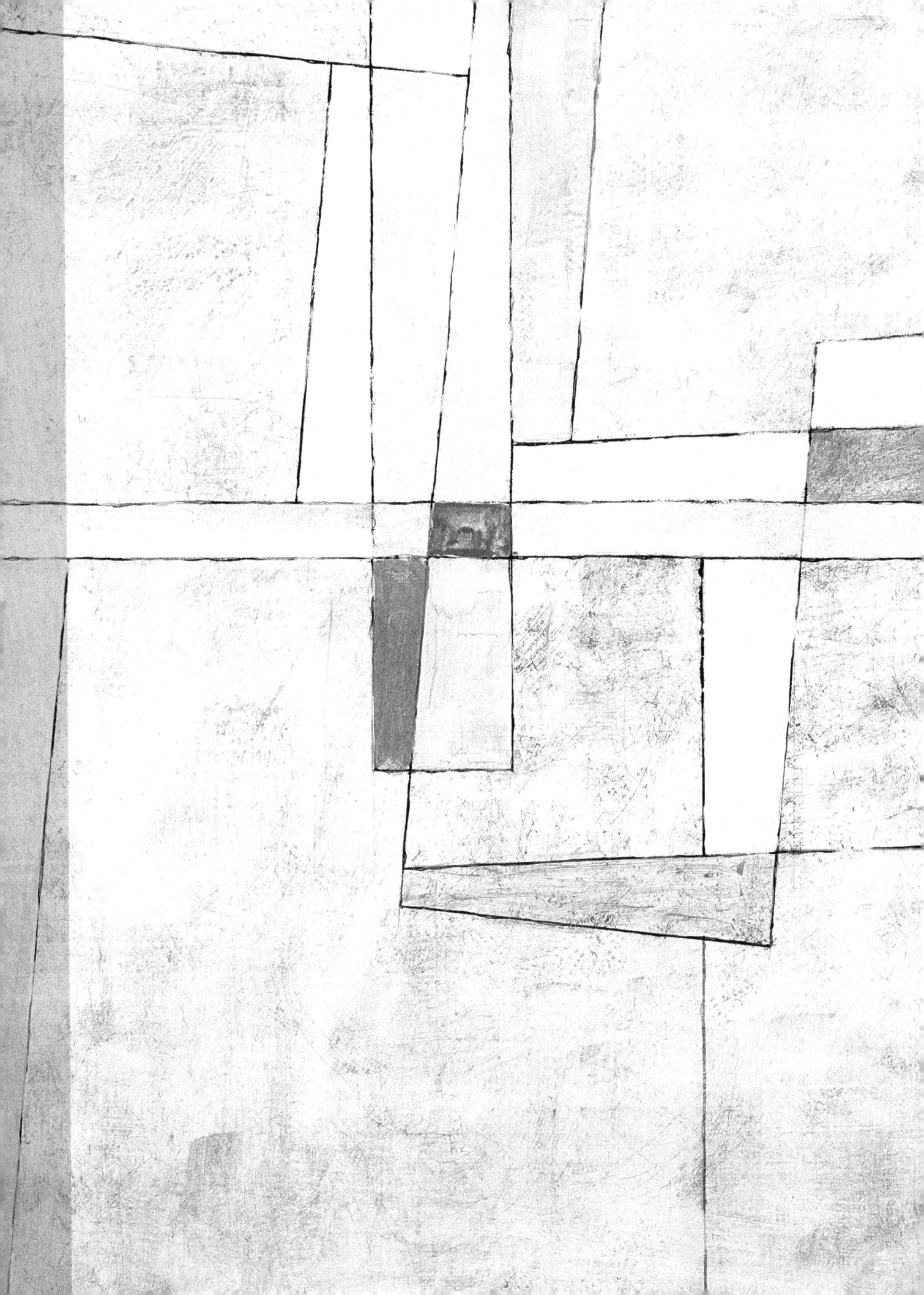

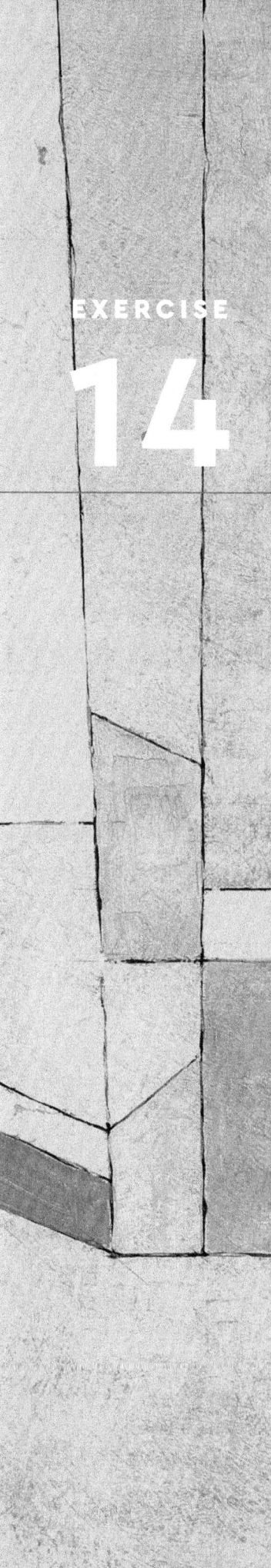

Mock Rational Emotive Behavior Therapy Sessions

In contrast to highly structured and repetitive deliberate practice exercises, a mock rational emotive behavior therapy (REBT) session is an unstructured and improvised role-play therapy session. Like a jazz rehearsal, mock sessions let you practice the art and science of *appropriate responsiveness* (Hatcher, 2015; Stiles & Horvath, 2017), putting your psychotherapy skills together in a way that is helpful to your mock client. This exercise outlines the procedure for conducting a mock REBT session. It offers different client profiles you may choose to adopt when enacting with a client.

Mock sessions are an opportunity for trainees to practice the following:

- using psychotherapy skills responsively
- navigating challenging choice-points in therapy
- choosing which interventions to use
- tracking the arc of a therapy session and the overall big-picture therapy treatment
- guiding treatment in the context of the client's preferences
- determining realistic goals for therapy in the context of the client's capacities
- knowing how to proceed when the therapist is unsure, lost, or confused
- recognizing and recovering from therapeutic errors
- discovering your personal therapeutic style
- building endurance for working with real clients

Mock REBT Session Overview

For the mock session, **you will perform a role-play of an initial therapy session**. As is true with the exercises to build individual skills, the role-play involves three people: One trainee role-plays the therapist, another trainee role-plays the client, and a trainer (a professor or a supervisor) observes and provides feedback. This is an open-ended role-play, as is commonly done in training. However, this differs in two important ways from the role-plays used in more traditional training. First, the therapist will use their

https://doi.org/10.1037/0000334–016

Deliberate Practice in Rational Emotive Behavior Therapy, by M. D. Terjesen, K. A. Doyle, R. A. DiGiuseppe, A. Vaz, and T. Rousmaniere

hand to indicate how difficult the role-play feels. Second, the client will attempt to make the role-play easier or harder to ensure the therapist is practicing at the right difficulty level.

Preparation

1. Download the Deliberate Practice Reaction Form and the Deliberate Practice Diary Form from the "Clinician and Practitioner Resources" tab at https://www.apa.org/pubs/books/deliberate-practice-rational-emotive-behavior-therapy (also available in Appendixes A and B, respectively). Every student will need their own copy of the Deliberate Practice Reaction Form on a separate piece of paper so that they can access it quickly.

2. Designate one student to role-play the therapist and one student to role-play the client. The trainer will observe and provide corrective feedback.

Mock REBT Session Procedure

1. The trainees will role-play an initial (first) therapy session. The trainee role-playing the client selects a client profile from the end of this exercise.

2. Before beginning the role-play, the therapist raises their hand to their side, at the level of their chair seat (see Figure E14.1). They will use this hand throughout the whole role-play to indicate how challenging it feels to them to help the client. Their starting hand level (chair seat) indicates that the role-play feels easy. By raising their hand, the

FIGURE E14.1. Ongoing Difficulty Assessment Through Hand Level

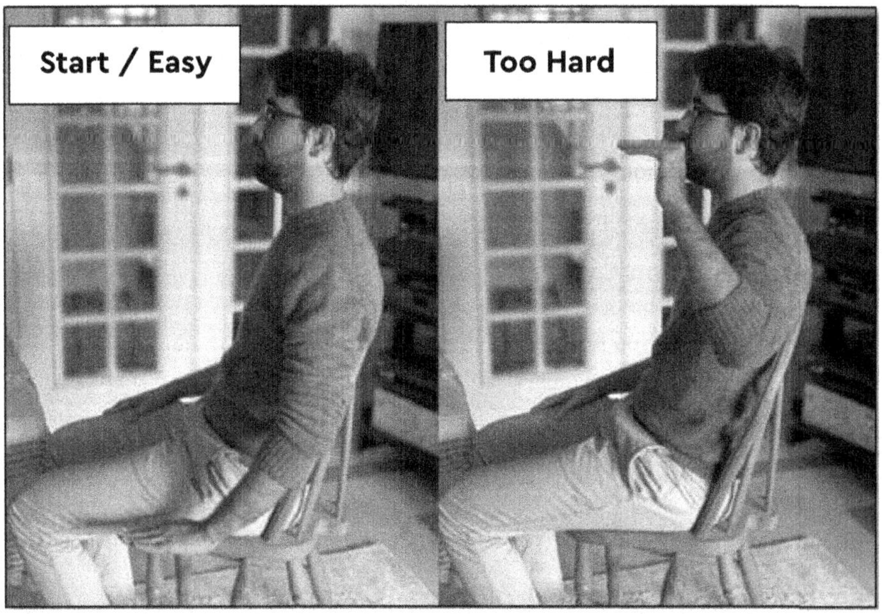

Note. Left: Start of role-play. Right: Role-play is too difficult. From *Deliberate Practice in Emotion-Focused Therapy* (p. 156), by R. N. Goldman, A. Vaz, and T. Rousmaniere, 2021, American Psychological Association (https://doi.org/10.1037/0000227-000). Copyright 2021 by the American Psychological Association.

therapist indicates that the difficulty is rising. If their hand rises above their neck level, it indicates that the role-play is too difficult.

3. The therapist begins the role-play. The therapist and client should engage in the role-play in an improvised manner, as they would engage in a real therapy session. The therapist keeps their hand out at their side throughout this process. (This may feel strange at first!)

4. Whenever the therapist feels that the difficulty of the role-play has changed significantly, they should move their hand up if it feels more difficult; down if it feels easier. If the therapist's hand drops below the seat of their chair, the client should make the role-play more challenging; if the therapist's hand rises above their neck level, the client should make the role-play easier. Instructions for adjusting the difficulty of the role-play are described in the "Varying the Level of Challenge" section.

Note to Therapists

Remember to be aware of your vocal quality. Match your tone to the client's presentation. Thus, if the clients present vulnerable, soft emotions behind their words, soften your tone to be soothing and calm. If clients, on the other hand, are aggressive and angry, match your tone to be firm and solid.

---

5. The role-play continues for at least 15 minutes. The trainer may provide corrective feedback during this process if the therapist gets significantly off-track. However, trainers should exercise restraint and keep feedback as short and tight as possible because this will reduce the therapist's opportunity for experiential training.

6. After the role-play is finished, the therapist and client switch roles and begin a new mock session.

7. After both trainees have completed the mock session as a therapist, the trainees and the trainer discuss the experience.

Varying the Level of Challenge

If the therapist indicates that the mock session is too easy, the person enacting the role of the client can use the following modifications to make it more challenging (see also Appendix A):

- The client can improvise with topics that are more evocative or make the therapist uncomfortable, such as expressing currently held strong feelings (see Figure A.2).

- The client can use a distressed voice (e.g., angry, sad, sarcastic) or unpleasant facial expression. This increases the emotional tone.

- Blend complex mixtures of opposing feelings (e.g., love and rage).

- Become confrontational, questioning the purpose of therapy or the therapist's fitness for the role.

If the therapist indicates that the mock session is too hard:

- The client can be guided by Figure A.2 to
  - present topics that are less evocative,
  - present material on any topic but without expressing feelings, or
  - present material concerning the future or the past or events outside therapy.

- The client can ask the questions in a soft voice or with a smile. This softens the emotional stimulus.

- The therapist can take short breaks during the role-play.

- The trainer can expand the "feedback phase" by discussing REBT or psychotherapy theory.

Mock Session Client Profiles

Following are six client profiles for trainees to use during mock sessions, presented in order of difficulty. The choice of client profile may be determined by the trainee playing the therapist, the trainee playing the client, or assigned by the trainer.

The most important aspect of role-plays is for trainees to convey the emotional tone indicated by the client profile (e.g., "angry," "sad"). The demographics of the client (e.g., age, gender) and specific content of the client profiles are not important. Thus, trainees should adjust the client profile to most comfortable and easy for the trainee to role-play. For example, a trainee may change the client profile from female to male, from 45 to 22 years old, and so on.

Beginner Profile: Processing Grief With a Receptive Client

Laura is a 28-year-old Latinx waitress whose mother died from cancer about 6 months ago. Laura has been experiencing sadness about losing her mother. She reports that sometimes her sadness is so debilitating that she withdraws from others and goes into "shutdown from life" mode. Of her emotions, she reports her grief is the most problematic. Laura's grief is complicated by feelings of anger she has about her mother not being very attentive or loving during Laura's childhood. She would often comment that she knew that her mother was very busy when she was growing up, caring for the family while trying to hold multiple jobs; however, Laura still believes that her mother was hard on her and that she should not have treated her the way that she did. Laura also misses her two siblings, who were forced to go back to Mexico because they were undocumented. Laura reports thinking that she is all alone now and that she can't handle these feelings. Laura wants help processing her grief and anger about her mother.

- **Symptoms:** Grief, anger, and loneliness

- **Client's goals for therapy:** Laura wants to process her complex feelings about her mother and reconnect with her siblings.

- **Attitude toward therapy:** Laura had good experiences in therapy previously when she was in high school and is optimistic about therapy helping again.

- **Strengths:** Laura is very motivated for therapy and is emotionally open with the therapist.

Beginner Profile: Addressing Loneliness With a Motivated Client

Susan is a 25-year-old African American accountant who recently moved across the country for a new job. While she loves her new job, she has had trouble making friends. She is coming to therapy because she is feeling lonely. She reported that she tries to journal daily, and when she does, she finds herself crying and lamenting about her life. She recently went on a date and was disappointed when it didn't go well. She's worried that she will get demoralized and stop trying to make new friends. She canceled plans for this weekend, and although she wants to be in a relationship, she sees the process of getting there as too difficult. She wonders if there is something inherently flawed about her because she has such difficulties making friends and when she looks at her life, she sees it as one that is empty and that is too much to bear.

- **Symptoms:** Loneliness, sadness, and demoralization

- **Client's goals for therapy:** Susan wants to build motivation to make more friends and go on more dates.

- **Attitude toward therapy:** Susan has had positive experiences in therapy before. She is hopeful that this therapy will help as well.

- **Strengths:** Susan is emotionally open and motivated to engage in the therapy tasks.

Intermediate Profile: Addressing Anxiety With a Nervous Client

Bob is a 35-year-old European American electrician who suffers from extreme anxiety, panic attacks, and shame. He feels like he has been a "loser" his whole life. He was bullied in high school and thinks that people still judge him. He tries to avoid contact with people except through online computer games. He reports that online people are nicer and that when he gets rejected in person, it is terrible. He was referred to therapy by his boss, who noticed that Bob would sometimes not show up for work or leave work early. Bob acknowledges this and reports that he thinks he couldn't deal with screwing up in front of others, and this would only confirm his status as a loser. Bob has trouble identifying any of his feelings except anxiety.

- **Symptoms:** Anxiety, panic attacks, and social isolation

- **Client's goals for therapy:** Bob wants to feel more confident socially so he can engage in work more reliably.

- **Attitude toward therapy:** Bob didn't want to come to therapy because he felt very nervous about it and thinks that the therapist will judge him. Bob's boss convinced him to try therapy.

- **Strengths:** Underneath his anxiety and shame, Bob really wants to connect with other people, including the therapist.

Intermediate Profile: Helping a Sarcastic and Skeptical Client

Jeff is a 45-year-old Asian American engineer who was referred to therapy by his employer because he has been getting angry at work. He is very smart and gets frustrated quickly when his colleagues do not understand his decisions. He reports that he is the smartest guy in the room and that they should not question what he does. When he gets frustrated, Jeff is sarcastic or mean. He communicated that he received a negative evaluation by his supervisor in the area of "team player," and he struggled to let that go.

Jeff understands that this is a problem and wants to be more friendly, but he has been unable to change his behavior. He knows that his colleagues do not like him, so he feels socially isolated at work.

- **Symptoms:** Outbursts of sarcasm and meanness that cover underlying loneliness and social isolation

- **Client's goals for therapy:** Jeff wants to learn how to be more patient and relate better to his colleagues.

- **Attitude toward therapy:** Jeff has never been in therapy before and is skeptical whether it will help. He came to therapy because his employer asked him to.

- **Strengths:** Jeff honestly wants to be more prosocial.

Advanced Profile: Helping a Very Distrustful Client With a History of Abuse and Discrimination

Betty is a 27-year-old African American graduate student in law school. She wants to become a public defender when she graduates. Betty is the oldest of four siblings. She and her siblings were sexually and physically abused by her father when she was a child. Her father also beat her mother frequently. (Her father is currently in prison for the physical and sexual abuse.) She also feels she has been very hurt and traumatized by systemic racism and discrimination. She has worked very hard to achieve her current status. She does not generally trust the system because she has not felt her interests have been prioritized or protected. Betty feels a lot of anger toward her father, and also toward her mother for not protecting her and her siblings. Her youngest sister recently committed suicide due to the abuse. Betty feels very guilty about not protecting her siblings from her father, and although she has both anger and guilt, she mostly wants to work on the overwhelming guilt she experiences. She has communicated that "I should have protected them back then, and I should have been more in tune with what my sister experienced and prevented her from committing suicide."

- **Symptoms:** Anger at parents, guilt about not protecting siblings, and grief about her sister's suicide

- **Client's goals for therapy:** Betty wants to resolve her guilt about her sister.

- **Attitude toward therapy:** Betty went to therapy in grade school but had a bad experience. When she told her therapist about her father's abuse, the therapist didn't believe her and told the father what Betty had said. (Betty found out later that the therapist was a friend of her father.) Thus, Betty is very distrustful of therapists, particular non–African American therapists.

- **Strengths:** Betty is focused and dedicated to improving her mental health. Betty is extremely resilient. She has strong convictions about social justice. She is fiercely loyal to her friends and family.

Advanced Profile: Helping a Client With Mood Lability and Who Self-Harms

Jane is a 20-year-old European American college student who is having problems in her relationship where she cycles between being deeply in love with her boyfriend and then hating him when he does something that disappoints her, like forgetting her birthday. When Jane is disappointed by her boyfriend, she feels betrayed and abandoned, gets very angry and depressed, and cuts herself. She reported at intake that "I have one birthday a year, he should have remembered that. Maybe because he didn't, it proves that I am not worthy of anyone." Jane has a similar pattern with her family and friends, where she cycles between liking them a lot and then feeling betrayed and abandoned when they disappoint her. She has indicated that being disappointed by those she trusts is the worst thing that could happen to her.

- **Symptoms:** Mood lability, self-harm (cutting), and relationship instability

- **Client's goals for therapy:** Jane wants to find stability in herself and her relationships.

- **Attitude toward therapy:** Jane was in therapy before, which was helpful until the therapist disappointed Jane by missing a session, after which Jane felt betrayed and abandoned and quit therapy. Jane is worried that you (her new therapist) may betray or abandon her.

- **Strengths:** Jane is very open to what the therapist says (when she feels safe in therapy).

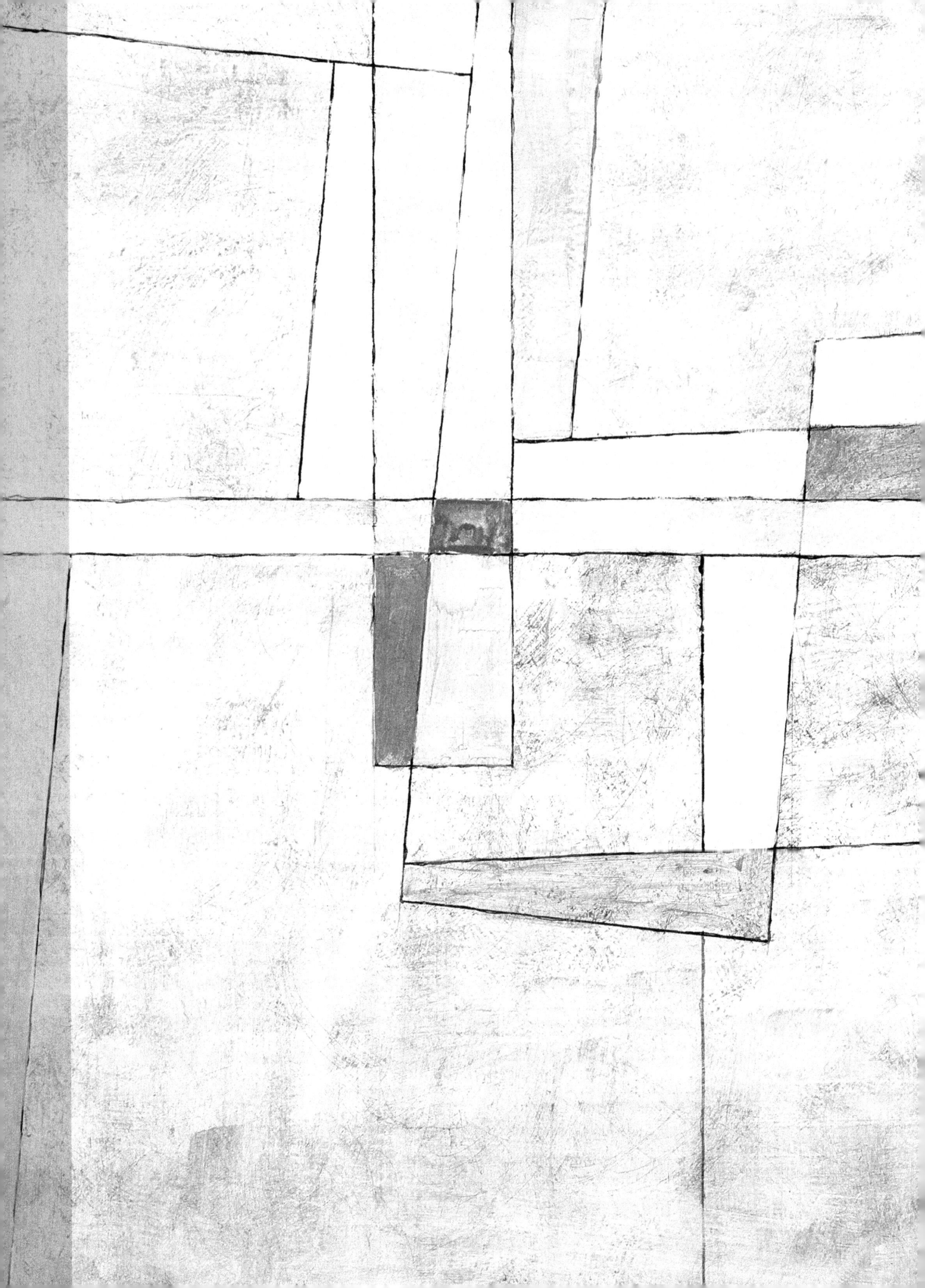

Strategies for Enhancing the Deliberate Practice Exercises

Part III consists of one chapter, Chapter 3, that provides additional advice and instructions for trainers and trainees so that they can reap more benefits from the deliberate practice exercises in Part II. Chapter 3 offers six key points for getting the most out of deliberate practice, guidelines for practicing appropriately responsive treatment, evaluation strategies, methods for ensuring trainee well-being and respecting their privacy, and advice for monitoring the trainer–trainee relationship.

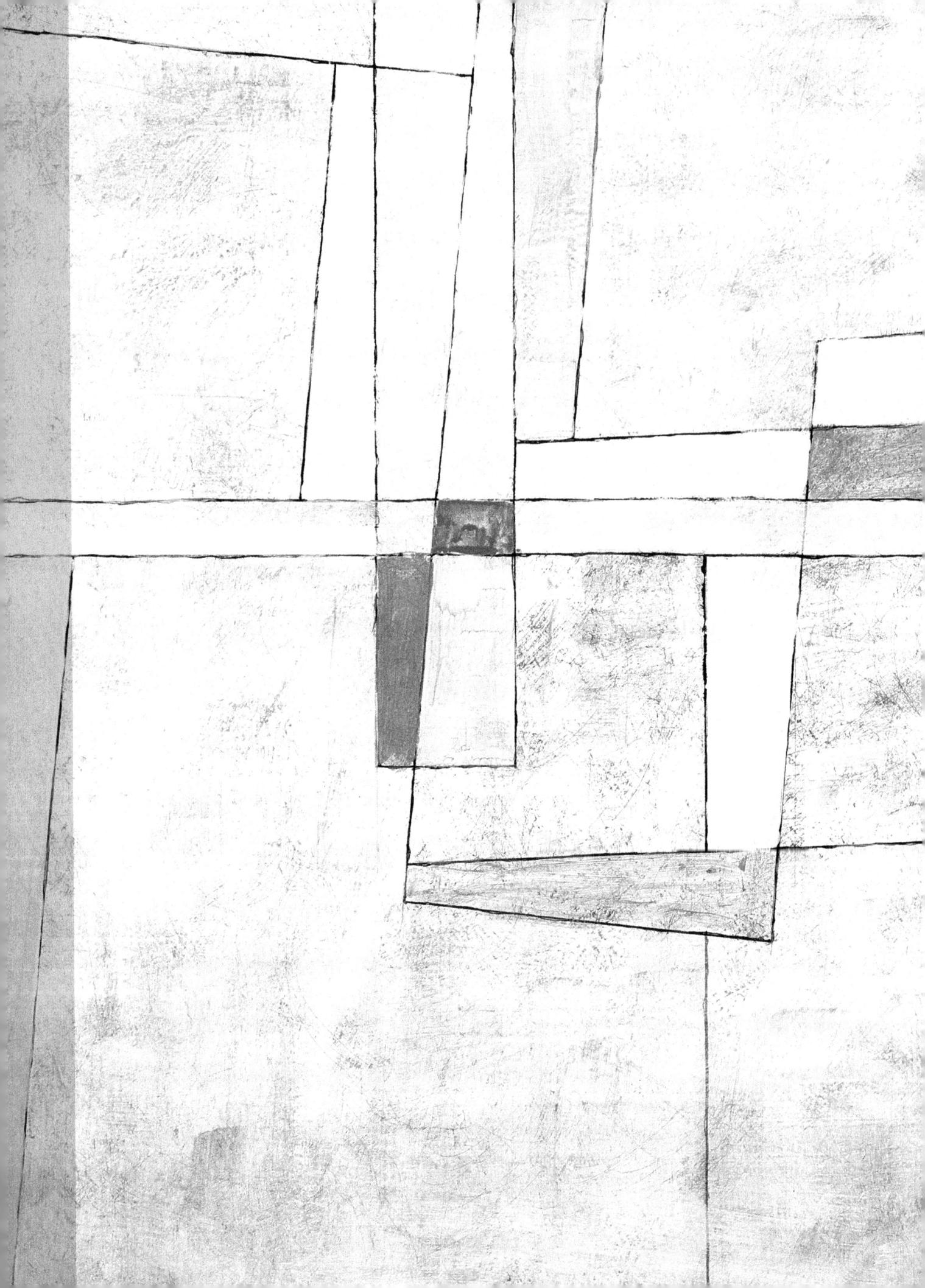

How to Get the Most Out of Deliberate Practice: Additional Guidance for Trainers and Trainees

In Chapter 2 and in the exercises themselves, we provide instructions for completing the deliberate practice exercises. This chapter provides guidance on big-picture topics that trainers will need to successfully integrate deliberate practice into their training program. This guidance is based on relevant research and the experiences and feedback from trainers at more than a dozen psychotherapy training programs who volunteered to test the deliberate practice exercises in this book. We cover topics including evaluation, getting the most from deliberate practice, trainee well-being, respecting trainee privacy, trainer self-evaluation, responsive treatment, and the trainee–trainer alliance.

Six Key Points for Getting the Most From Deliberate Practice

Following are six key points of advice for trainers and trainees to get the most benefit from the rational emotive behavior therapy (REBT) deliberate practice exercises. The following advice is gleaned from experiences vetting and practicing the exercises, sometimes in different languages, with many trainees, across many countries.

Key Point 1: Create Realistic Stimuli

A key component of deliberate practice is using stimuli that provoke similar reactions to challenging real-life work settings. For example, pilots train with flight simulators that present mechanical failures and dangerous weather conditions; surgeons practice with surgical simulators that present medical complications with only seconds to respond. Training with challenging stimuli will increase trainees' capacity to perform therapy effectively under stress—for example, with clients they find challenging. The stimuli used for REBT deliberate practice exercises are role-plays of challenging client statements in therapy. **It is important that the trainee who is role-playing the client perform the script with appropriate emotional expression and maintain eye contact with the**

https://doi.org/10.1037/0000334-017

Deliberate Practice in Rational Emotive Behavior Therapy, by M. D. Terjesen, K. A. Doyle, R. A. DiGiuseppe, A. Vaz, and T. Rousmaniere

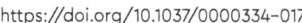

therapist. For example, if the client statement calls for sad emotion, the trainee should try to express sadness eye-to-eye with the therapist. We offer the following suggestions regarding emotional expressiveness:

1. The emotional tone of the role-play matters more than the exact words of each script. Trainees role-playing the client should feel free to improvise and change the words if it will help them be more emotionally expressive, but when the skill calls for demonstration of a clinical response to specific irrational belief(s), the clients are encouraged to present those specific belief(s). Trainees do not need to stick 100% exactly to the script. In fact, to read off the script during the exercise can sound flat and prohibit eye contact. Rather, trainees in the client role should first read the client statement silently to themselves, then, when ready, say it in an emotional manner while looking directly at the trainee playing the therapist. This will help the experience feel more real and engaging for the therapist.

2. Trainees whose first language isn't English may particularly benefit from reviewing and changing the words in the client statement script before each role-play so they can find words that feel congruent and facilitate emotional expression.

3. Trainees role-playing the client should try to use tonal and nonverbal expressions of feelings. For example, if a script calls for anger, the trainee can speak with an angry voice and make fists with their hands; if a script calls for shame or guilt, the trainee could hunch over and wince; if a script calls for sadness, the trainee could speak in a soft or deflated voice.

4. If trainees are having persistent difficulties acting believably when following a particular script in the role of client, it may help to first do a "demo round" by reading directly from paper, and then, immediately after, dropping the paper to make eye contact and repeating the same client statement from memory. Some trainees reported this helped them "become available as real clients" and made the role-play feel less artificial. Some trainees did three or four "demo rounds" to get fully into their role as a client.

Key Point 2: Customize the Exercises to Fit Your Unique Training Circumstances

Deliberate practice is less about adhering to specific rules than it is about using training principles. Every trainer has their own individual teaching style and every trainee their own learning process. Thus, the exercises in this book are designed to be flexibly customized by trainers across different training contexts within different cultures. Trainees and trainers are encouraged to continually adjust exercises to optimize their practice. The most effective training will occur when deliberate practice exercises are customized to fit the learning needs of each trainee and culture of each training site. In our experience with numerous trainers and trainees across many countries, we found that everyone spontaneously customized the exercises for their unique training circumstances. No two trainers followed the exact same procedure. For example:

- One supervisor used the exercises with a trainee who found all the client statements to be too hard, including the "beginner" stimuli. This trainee had multiple reactions in the "too hard" category, including nausea, severe shame, and self-doubt. The trainee disclosed to the supervisor that she had experienced extremely harsh learning environments earlier in her life and found the role-plays to be highly evocative. To help, the supervisor followed the suggestions offered in Appendix A to make the stimuli progressively easier until the trainee reported feeling "good challenge" on the Deliberate Practice Reaction Form. Over many weeks of practice, the trainee developed a sense of safety and was able to practice with more difficult client statements. (Note that if the supervisor had proceeded at the "too hard" difficulty level, the trainee might have complied while hiding her negative reactions, become emotionally flooded and overwhelmed, leading to withdrawal and thus prohibiting her skill development and risking dropout from training.)

- Supervisors of trainees for whom English was not their first language adjusted the client statements to their own primary language.

- One supervisor used the exercises with a trainee who found all the stimuli to be too easy, including the advanced client statements. This supervisor quickly moved to improvising more challenging client statements from scratch by following the instructions in Appendix A on how to make client statements more challenging.

Key Point 3: Discover Your Own Unique Personal Therapeutic Style

Deliberate practice in psychotherapy can be likened to the process of learning to play jazz music. Every jazz musician prides themselves in their skillful improvisations, and the process of "finding your own voice" is a prerequisite for expertise in jazz musicianship. Yet, improvisations are not a collection of random notes but the culmination of extensive deliberate practice over time. Indeed, the ability to improvise is built upon many hours of dedicated practice of scales, melodies, harmonies, and so on. In much the same way, psychotherapy trainees are encouraged to experience the scripted interventions in this book not as ends in themselves but to promote skill in a systematic fashion. Over time, effective therapeutic creativity can be aided, instead of constrained, by dedicated practice in these therapeutic "melodies."

Key Point 4: Engage in a Sufficient Amount of Rehearsal

Deliberate practice uses rehearsal to move skills into procedural memory, which helps trainees maintain access to skills even when working with challenging clients. This only works if trainees engage in many repetitions of the exercises. Think of a challenging sport or musical instrument you learned: How many rehearsals would a professional need to feel confident performing a new skill? Psychotherapy is no easier than those other fields!

Key Point 5: Continually Adjust Difficulty

A crucial element of deliberate practice is training at an optimal difficulty level: neither too easy nor too hard. To achieve this, do difficulty assessments and adjustments with the Deliberate Practice Reaction Form in Appendix A. **Do not skip this step!** If trainees don't feel any of the "good challenge" reactions at the bottom of the Deliberate Practice Reaction Form, then the exercise is probably too easy; if they feel any of the "too hard" reactions, then the exercise could be too difficult for the trainee to benefit. Advanced trainees and therapists may find all the client statements too easy. If so, they should follow the instructions in Appendix A on making client statements harder to make the role-plays sufficiently challenging.

Key Point 6: Putting It All Together With the Practice Transcript and Mock Therapy Sessions

Some trainees may feel a further need for greater contextualization of the individual therapy responses associated with each skill, feeling the need to integrate the disparate pieces of their training in a more coherent manner, with a simulation that mimics a real therapy session. The annotated transcript in Exercise 13 and the mock therapy sessions in Exercise 14 give trainees this opportunity, allowing them to practice delivering different responses sequentially in a more realistic therapeutic encounter.

Responsive Treatment

The exercises in this book are designed to help trainees not only acquire specific skills of REBT but also use them in ways that are responsive to each individual client. Across the psychotherapy literature, this stance has been referred to as *appropriate responsiveness*, wherein the therapists exercise flexible judgment, based on their perception of the client's emotional state, needs, and goals, and integrate techniques and other interpersonal skills in pursuit of optimal client outcomes (Hatcher, 2015; Stiles et al., 1998). The effective therapist is responsive to the emerging context. As Stiles and Horvath (2017) argued, a therapist is effective because they are appropriately responsive. Doing the "right thing" may be different each time and means providing each client with an individually tailored response.

Appropriate responsiveness counters a misconception that deliberate practice rehearsal is designed to promote robotic repetition of therapy techniques. Psychotherapy researchers have shown that overadherence to a particular model while neglecting client preferences reduces therapy effectiveness (e.g., Castonguay et al., 1996; Henry et al., 1993; Owen & Hilsenroth, 2014). Therapist flexibility, on the other hand, has been shown to improve outcomes (e.g., Bugatti & Boswell, 2016; Kendall & Beidas, 2007; Kendall & Frank, 2018). It is important, therefore, that trainees practice their newly learned skills in a manner that is flexible and responsive to the unique needs of a diverse range of clients (Hatcher, 2015; Hill & Knox, 2013). It is of paramount importance for trainees to develop the necessary perceptual skills to be attuned to what the client is experiencing in the moment and form their response based on the client moment-by-moment context.

It is also important that deliberate practice occurs within a context of wider REBT learning. As noted in Chapter 1, training should be combined with supervision of actual therapy recordings, theoretical learning, observation of competent REBT psychotherapists, and personal therapeutic work. When the trainer or trainee determines that the trainee is having difficulty acquiring REBT skills, it is important to carefully assess what is missing or needed. Assessment should then lead to the appropriate remedy, as the trainer and trainee collaboratively determine what is needed.

Being Mindful of Trainee Well-Being

Although the negative effects that some clients experience in psychotherapy have been well documented (Barlow, 2010), negative effects of training and supervision on trainees have received less attention (M. V. Ellis et al., 2014). To support strong self-efficacy, trainers must ensure that trainees are practicing at a correct difficulty level. The exercises in this book feature guidance for frequently assessing and adjusting the difficulty level, so trainees can rehearse at a level that precisely targets their personal skill threshold. Trainers and supervisors must be mindful to provide an appropriate challenge. One risk to trainees that is particularly pertinent to this book occurs when using role-plays that are too difficult. The Deliberate Practice Reaction Form in Appendix A is provided to help trainers ensure that role-plays are done at an appropriate challenge level. Trainers or trainees may be tempted to skip the difficulty assessments and adjustments, out of their motivation to focus on rehearsal in order to make fast progress and quickly acquire skills. But across all our test sites, we found that skipping the difficulty assessments and adjustments caused more problems and hindered skill acquisition more than any other error. Thus, trainers are advised to remember that **one of their most important responsibilities is to remind trainees to do the difficulty assessments and adjustments**.

Additionally, the Reaction Form serves a dual purpose of helping trainees develop the important skills of self-monitoring and self-awareness (Bennett-Levy, 2019). This will help trainees adopt a positive and empowered stance regarding their own self-care and should facilitate career-long professional development.

Respecting Trainee Privacy

The deliberate practice exercises in this book may stir up complex or uncomfortable personal reactions in trainees, including, for example, memories of past traumas. Exploring psychological and emotional reactions may make some trainees feel vulnerable. Therapists at every career stage, from trainees to seasoned therapists with decades of experience, commonly experience shame, embarrassment, and self-doubt in this process. Although these experiences can be valuable for building trainees' self-awareness, it is important that training remain focused on professional skill development and not blur into personal therapy (e.g., M. V. Ellis et al., 2014). Therefore, one trainer role is to remind trainees to maintain appropriate boundaries.

Trainees must have the final say about what to disclose or not disclose to their trainer. Trainees should keep in mind that the goal is for the trainee to expand their own self-awareness and psychological capacity to stay active and helpful while experiencing uncomfortable reactions. The trainer does not need to know the specific details about the trainee's inner world for this to happen.

Trainees should be instructed to share only personal information that they feel comfortable sharing. The Reaction Form and difficulty assessment process are designed to help trainees build their self-awareness while retaining control over their privacy. Trainees can be reminded that the goal is for them to learn about their own inner world. They do not necessarily have to share that information with trainers or peers (Bennett-Levy & Finlay-Jones, 2018). Likewise, trainees should be instructed to respect the confidentiality of their peers.

Trainer Self-Evaluation

The exercises in this book were tested at a wide range of training sites around the world, including graduate courses, practicum sites, and private practice offices. Although trainers reported that the exercises were highly effective for training, some also said that they felt disoriented by how different deliberate practice feels compared with their traditional methods of clinical education. Many felt comfortable evaluating their trainees' performance but were less sure about their own performance as trainers.

The most common concern we heard from trainers was, "My trainees are doing great, but I'm not sure if I am doing this correctly!" To address this concern, we recommend trainers perform periodic self-evaluations along the following five criteria:

1. Observe trainees' work performance.
2. Provide continual corrective feedback.
3. Ensure rehearsal of specific skills is just beyond the trainees' current ability.
4. Ensure that the trainee is practicing at the right difficulty level (neither too easy nor too challenging).
5. Continuously assess trainee performance with real clients.

Criterion 1: Observe Trainees' Work Performance

Determining how well we are doing as trainers means first having valid information about how well trainees are responding to training. This requires that we directly observe trainees practicing skills in order to provide corrective feedback and evaluation. One risk of deliberate practice is that trainees gain competence in performing therapy skills in role-plays, but those skills do not transfer to trainees' work with real clients. Thus, trainers will ideally also have the opportunity to observe samples of trainees' work with real clients, either live or via recorded video. Supervisors and consultants rely heavily—and, too often, exclusively—on supervisees' and consultees' narrative accounts of their work with clients (Goodyear & Nelson, 1997). Haggerty and Hilsenroth (2011) described this challenge:

> Suppose a loved one has to undergo surgery and you need to choose between two surgeons, one of whom has never been directly observed by an experienced surgeon while performing any surgery. He or she would perform the surgery and return to his or her attending physician and try to recall, sometimes incompletely or inaccurately, the intricate steps of the surgery they just performed. It is hard to imagine that anyone, given a choice, would prefer this over a professional who has been routinely observed in the practice of their craft. (p. 193)

Criterion 2: Provide Continual Corrective Feedback

Trainees need corrective feedback to learn what they are doing well, what they are doing poorly, and how to improve their skills. Feedback should be as specific and incremental as possible. Examples of specific feedback are, "Your voice sounds rushed. Try slowing down by pausing for a few seconds between your statements to the client," and, "That's excellent how you are making eye contact with the client." Examples of vague and nonspecific feedback are, "Try to build better rapport with the client," and, "Try to be more open to the client's feelings."

Criterion 3: Specific Skill Rehearsal Just Beyond the Trainees' Current Ability (Zone of Proximal Development)

Deliberate practice emphasizes skill acquisition via behavioral rehearsal. Trainers should endeavor to not get caught up in client conceptualization at the expense of focusing on skills. For many trainers, this requires significant discipline and self-restraint. It is simply more enjoyable to talk about psychotherapy theory (e.g., case conceptualization, treatment planning, nuances of psychotherapy models, similar cases the supervisor has had) than watch trainees rehearse skills. Trainees have many questions and supervisors have an abundance of experience; the allotted supervision time can easily be filled by sharing knowledge. The supervisor gets to sound smart, while the trainee doesn't have to struggle with acquiring skills at their learning edge. While answering questions is important, trainees' intellectual knowledge about psychotherapy can quickly surpass their procedural ability to perform psychotherapy, particularly with clients they find challenging. Here's a simple rule of thumb: The trainer provides the knowledge, but the behavioral rehearsal provides the skill (Rousmaniere, 2019).

Criterion 4: Practice at the Right Difficulty Level (Neither Too Easy nor Too Challenging)

Deliberate practice involves *optimal strain*: practicing skills just beyond the trainee's current skill threshold so they can learn incrementally without becoming overwhelmed (Ericsson, 2006).

Trainers should use difficulty assessments and adjustments throughout deliberate practice to ensure that trainees are practicing at the right difficulty level. Note that some trainees are surprised by their unpleasant reactions to exercises (e.g., disassociation, nausea, blanking out), and may be tempted to "push through" exercises that are too hard. This can happen out of fear of failing a course, fear of being judged as incompetent, or negative self-impressions by the trainee (e.g., "This shouldn't be so hard"). Trainers should normalize the fact that there will be wide variation in perceived difficulty of the exercises and encourage trainees to respect their own personal training process.

Criterion 5: Continuously Assess Trainee Performance With Real Clients

The goal of deliberately practicing psychotherapy skills is to improve trainees' effectiveness at helping real clients. One of the risks in deliberate practice training is that the benefits will not generalize: Trainees' acquired competence in specific skills may not translate into work with real clients. Thus, it is important that trainers assess the impact of deliberate practice on trainees' work with real clients. Ideally, this is done through triangulation of multiple data points:

1. client data (verbal self-report and routine outcome monitoring data)
2. supervisor's report
3. trainee's self-report

If the trainee's effectiveness with real clients is not improving after deliberate practice, the trainer should do a careful assessment of the difficulty. If the supervisor or trainer feels it is a skill acquisition issues, they may want to consider adjusting the deliberate practice routine to better suit the trainee's learning needs and/or style.

Therapists have traditionally been evaluated from a lens of *process accountability* (Markman & Tetlock, 2000; see also Goodyear, 2015), which focuses on demonstrating specific behaviors (e.g., fidelity to a treatment model) without regard to the impact on clients. We propose that clinical effectiveness is better assessed through a lens tightly focused on client outcomes and that learning objectives shift from performing behaviors that experts have decided are effective (i.e., the competence model) to highly individualized behavioral goals tailored to each trainee's zone of proximal development and performance feedback. This model of assessment has been termed *outcome accountability* (Goodyear, 2015), which focuses on client changes, rather than therapist competence, independent of how the therapist might be performing expected tasks.

Guidance for Trainees

The central theme of this book has been that skill rehearsal is not automatically helpful. Deliberate practice must be done well for trainees to benefit (Ericsson & Pool, 2016). In this chapter and in the exercises, we offer guidance for effective deliberate practice. We would also like to provide additional advice specifically for trainees. That advice is drawn from what we have learned at our volunteer deliberate practice test sites around the world. We cover how to discover your own training process, active effort, playfulness and taking breaks during deliberate practice, your right to control your self-disclosure to trainers, monitoring training results, monitoring complex reactions towards the trainer, and your own personal therapy.

Individualized REBT Training: Finding Your Zone of Proximal Development

Deliberate practice works best when training targets each trainee's personal skill thresholds. Also termed the *zone of proximal development*, a term first coined by Vygotsky in reference to developmental learning theory (Zaretskii, 2009), this is the area just beyond the trainee's current ability but which is possible to reach with the assistance of a teacher or coach (Wass & Golding, 2014). **If a deliberate practice exercise is either too easy or too hard, the trainee will not benefit.** To maximize training productivity, elite performers follow a "challenging but not overwhelming" principle: Tasks that are too far beyond their capacity will prove ineffective and even harmful; it is equally true that mindlessly repeating what they already can do confidently will prove fruitless. Because of this, deliberate practice requires ongoing assessment of the trainee's current skill and concurrent difficulty adjustment to consistently target a "good enough" challenge. Thus, if you are practicing Exercise 8, Functional Disputation of Irrational Beliefs, and it just feels too difficult, consider moving back to a more comfortable skill such as Exercise 4, Clarifying Inferences From Irrational Beliefs, or Exercise 5, Assessing Irrational Beliefs About the Activating Event, that they may feel they have already mastered.

Active Effort

It is important for trainees to maintain an active and sustained effort while doing the deliberate practice exercises in this book. Deliberate practice helps most when trainees push themselves up to and past their current ability. This is best achieved when trainees take ownership of their own practice by guiding their training partners to adjust role-plays to be as high on the difficulty scale as possible without hurting themselves. This will look different for every trainee. Although it can feel uncomfortable or even frightening, this is the zone of proximal development where the most gains can be made. Simply reading and repeating the written scripts will provide little or no benefit. Trainees are advised to remember that their effort from training should lead to more confidence and comfort in session with real clients.

Stay the Course: Effort Versus Flow

Deliberate practice works only if trainees push themselves hard enough to break out of their old patterns of performance, which then permits growth of new skills (Ericsson & Pool, 2016). Because deliberate practice constantly focuses on the current edge of one's performance capacity, it is inevitably a straining endeavor. Indeed, professionals are unlikely to make lasting performance improvements unless there is sufficient engagement in tasks that are just at the edge of one's current capacity (Ericsson, 2003,

2006). From athletics or fitness training, many of us are familiar with this process of being pushed out of our comfort zones followed by adaptation. The same process applies to our mental and emotional abilities.

Many trainees might feel surprised to discover that deliberate practice for REBT feels harder than psychotherapy with a real client. This may be because when working with a real client a therapist can get into a state of *flow* (Csikszentmihalyi, 1997), where work feels effortless. As a young REBT therapist in training, I (M.D.T.) was instructed not to engage in practical problem-solving (a skill that I believed that I was adept at) but focus on identifying, challenging, and changing irrational beliefs of clients (something that was a new language to me and I did not consider myself proficient at). As a result, I often felt frustrated after psychotherapy sessions. REBT therapists in training may find it difficult to teach the ABC model of REBT (Exercise 1) continually and believe that they are "just repeating themselves" or have captured the experience as best as they can and are ready to move forward. In such cases, therapists may want to move back to offering response formats with which they are more familiar and feel more proficient and try those for a short time, in part to increase a sense of confidence and mastery.

Discover Your Own Training Process

The effectiveness of deliberate practice is directly related to the effort and ownership trainees exert while doing the exercises. Trainers can provide guidance, but it is important for trainees to learn about their own idiosyncratic training processes over time. This will let them become masters of their own training and prepare for a career-long process of professional development. The following are a few examples of personal training processes trainees discovered while engaging in deliberate practice:

- One trainee noticed that she is good at persisting while an exercise is challenging, but also that she requires more rehearsal than other trainees to feel comfortable with a new skill. This trainee focused on developing patience with her own pace of progress.

- One trainee noticed that he can acquire new skills rather quickly, with only a few repetitions. However, he also noticed that his reactions to evocative client statements can jump very quickly and unpredictably from the "good challenge" to "too hard" categories, so he needs to carefully attend to the reactions listed in the Deliberate Practice Reaction Form.

- One trainee described herself as "perfectionistic" and felt a strong urge to "push through" an exercise even when she had anxiety reactions in the "too hard" category, such as nausea and disassociation. This caused the trainee not to benefit from the exercises and potentially become demoralized. This trainee focused on going slower, developing self-compassion regarding her anxiety reactions, and asking her training partners to make role-plays less challenging.

- One trainee reported greater comfort with the functional dispute (Exercise 8) and not the others in her clinical practice and believed that, although effective, she had come to rely too often on this one disputational strategy. This led to the trainee increasing the amount of time she focused on the other disputation skills (Exercises 9 and 10) and would seek specific feedback about her performance in these skills.

Trainees are encouraged to reflect deeply on their own experiences using the exercises to learn the most about themselves and their personal learning processes.

Playfulness and Taking Breaks

Psychotherapy is serious work that often involves painful feelings. However, practicing psychotherapy can be playful and fun (Scott Miller, personal communication, 2017). Trainees should remember that one of the main goals of deliberate practice is to experiment with different approaches and styles of therapy. If deliberate practice ever feels rote, boring, or routine, it probably isn't going to help advance trainees' skill. In this case, trainees should try to liven it up. A good way to do this is to introduce an atmosphere of playfulness. For example, trainees can try the following:

- Use different vocal tones, speech pacing, body gestures, or other languages. This can expand trainees' communication range.

- Practice while simulating being blind (with a cloth) or deaf. This can increase sensitivity in the other senses.

- Practice while standing up or walking around outside. This can help trainees get new perspectives on the process of therapy.

The supervisor can also ask trainees if they would like to take a 5- to 10-minute break between segments, particularly if the trainees are dealing with difficult emotions and are feeling stressed out.

Additional Deliberate Practice Opportunities

This book focuses on deliberate practice methods that involve active, live engagement between trainees and a supervisor. Importantly, deliberate practice can extend beyond these focused training sessions and be used for homework. For example, a trainee might read the client stimuli quietly or aloud and practice their responses independently between sessions with a supervisor. In such cases, it is important for the trainee to say their therapist responses aloud, rather than rehearse silently in one's head. Alternatively, two trainees can practice as a pair, without the supervisor. Although the absence of a supervisor limits one source of feedback, the peer trainee who is playing the client can serve this role, as they can when a supervisor is present. These additional deliberate practice opportunities are intended to take place between focused training sessions with a supervisor. To optimize the quality of the deliberate practice when conducted independently or without a supervisor, we have developed a Deliberate Practice Diary Form that can be found in Appendix B or downloaded from https://www.apa.org/pubs/books/deliberate-practice-rational-emotive-behavior-therapy (see the "Clinician and Practitioner Resources" tab). This form provides a template for the trainee to record their experience of the deliberate practice activity, and, ideally, it will aid in the consolidation of learning. This form can be used as part of the evaluation process with the supervisor, but it is not necessarily intended for that purpose, and trainees are certainly welcome to bring their experience with the independent practice into the next meeting with the supervisor.

Monitoring Training Results

While trainers will evaluate trainees using a competency-focused model, trainees are also encouraged to take ownership of their own training process and look for results of deliberate practice themselves. Trainees should experience the results of deliberate practice within a few training sessions. A lack of results can be demoralizing for trainees and can result in trainees applying less effort and focus in deliberate practice. Trainees who are not seeing results should openly discuss this problem with their trainer and experiment with adjusting their deliberate practice process. Results can include client outcomes and improving the trainee's own work as a therapist, their personal development, and their overall training.

Client Outcomes

The most important result of deliberate practice is an improvement in trainees' client outcomes. This can be assessed via routine outcome measurement (Lambert, 2010; Prescott et al., 2017), qualitative data (McLeod, 2017), and informal discussions with clients. However, trainees should note that an improvement in client outcome due to deliberate practice can sometimes be challenging to achieve quickly, given that the largest amount of variance in client outcome is due to client variables (Bohart & Wade, 2013). For example, a client with severe chronic symptoms may not respond quickly to any treatment, regardless of how effectively a trainee practices. For some clients, an increase in patience and self-compassion regarding their symptoms may be a sign of progress, rather than an immediate decrease in symptoms. Thus, trainees are advised to keep their expectations for client change realistic in the context of their client's symptoms, history, and presentation. It is important that trainees do not try to force their clients to improve in therapy in order for the former to feel like they are making progress in their training (Rousmaniere, 2016).

Trainee's Work as a Therapist

One important result of deliberate practice is change within the trainee regarding their work with clients. For example, trainees at test sites reported feeling more comfortable sitting with evocative clients, more confident addressing uncomfortable topics in therapy, and more responsive to a broader range of clients.

Trainee's Personal Development

Another important result of deliberate practice is personal growth within the trainee. For example, trainees at test sites reported becoming more in touch with their own feelings, increased self-compassion, and enhanced motivation to work with a broader range of clients.

Trainee's Training Process

Another valuable result of deliberate practice is improvement in the trainees' training process. For example, trainees at test sites reported becoming more aware of their personal training style, preferences, strengths, and challenges. Over time, trainees should grow to feel more ownership of their training process. It is also recommended that training to be a psychotherapist is a complex process that occurs over many years. Experienced, expert therapists still report continuing to grow well beyond their graduate school years (Orlinsky & Ronnestad, 2005).

The Trainee–Trainer Alliance: Monitoring Complex Reactions Toward the Trainer

Trainees who engage in hard deliberate practice often report experiencing complex feelings toward their trainer. For example, one trainee said, "I know this is helping, but I also don't look forward to it!" Another trainee reported feeling both appreciation and frustration towards her trainer simultaneously. Trainees are advised to remember intensive training they have done in other fields, such as athletics or music. When a coach pushes a trainee to the edge of their ability, it is common for trainees to have complex reactions toward them.

This does not necessarily mean that the trainer is doing anything wrong. In fact, intensive training inevitably stirs up reactions toward the trainer, such as frustration, annoyance, disappointment, or anger that coexist with the appreciations they feel. In fact, if trainees do not experience complex reactions, it is worth considering if the deliberate practice is sufficiently challenging. But what we asserted earlier about rights to privacy apply here as well. Because professional mental health training is hierarchical, and evaluative, trainers should not require or even expect trainees to share complex reactions they may be experiencing toward them. Trainers should stay open to their sharing, but the choice always remains with the trainee.

Trainee's Own Therapy

When engaging in deliberate practice, many trainees discover aspects of their inner world that may benefit from attending their own psychotherapy. For example, one trainee discovered that her clients' anger stirred up her own painful memories of abuse, another trainee found himself dissociating while practicing empathy skills, and another trainee experienced overwhelming shame and self-judgment when she couldn't master skills after just a few repetitions.

Although these discoveries were unnerving at first, they were ultimately beneficial because they motivated the trainees to seek out their own therapy. Many therapists attend their own therapy. In fact, Norcross and Guy (2005) found in their review of 17 studies that about 75% of the more than 8,000 therapist participants had attended their own therapy. Orlinsky and Ronnestad (2005) found that more than 90% of therapists who attended their own therapy reported it as helpful.

QUESTIONS FOR TRAINEES

1. Are you balancing the effort to improve your skills with patience and self-compassion for your learning process?
2. Are you attending to any shame or self-judgment that is arising from training?
3. Are you being mindful of your personal boundaries and also respecting any complex feelings you may have toward your trainers?

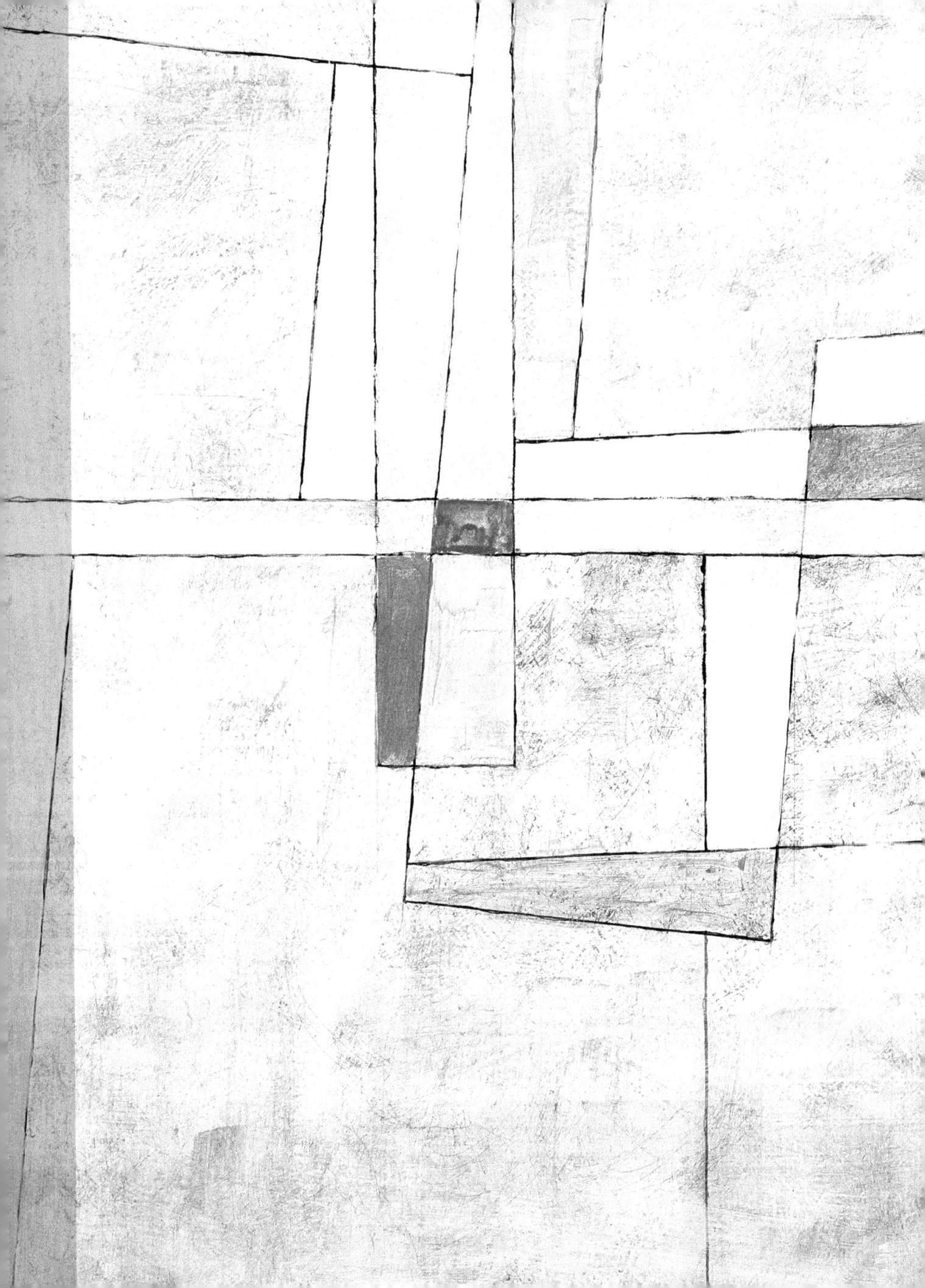

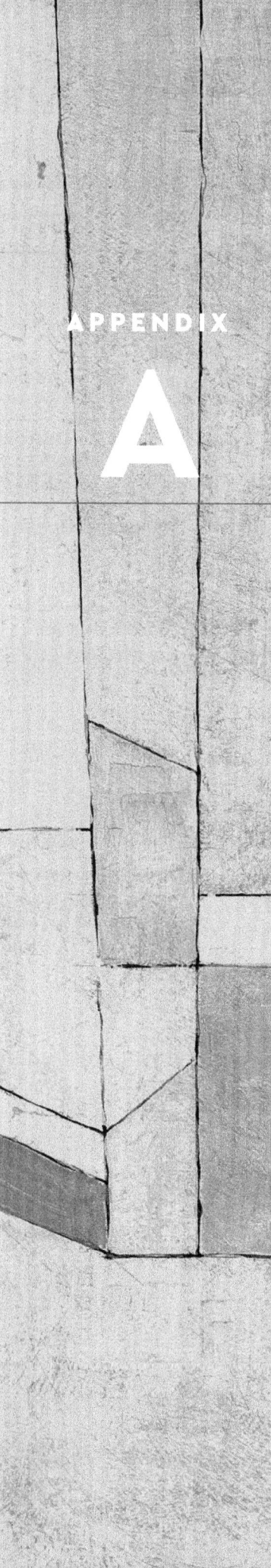

Difficulty Assessments
and Adjustments

Deliberate practice works best if the exercises are performed at a good challenge that is neither too hard nor too easy. To ensure that they are practicing at the correct difficulty, trainees should do a difficulty assessment and adjustment after each level of client statement is completed (beginner, intermediate, and advanced). To do this, use the following instructions and the Deliberate Practice Reaction Form (Figure A.1), which is also available in the "Clinician and Practitioner Resources" tab online (https://www.apa.org/pubs/books/deliberate-practice-rational-emotive-behavior-therapy). **Do not skip this process!**

How to Assess Difficulty

The therapist completes the Deliberate Practice Reaction Form (Figure A.1). If they

- rate the difficulty of the exercise above an 8 or had any of the reactions in the "Too Hard" column, follow the instructions to make the exercise easier;

- rate the difficulty of the exercise below a 4 or didn't have any of the reactions in the "Good Challenge" column, proceed to the next level of harder client statements or follow the instructions to make the exercise harder; or

- rate the difficulty of the exercise between 4 and 8 and have at least one reaction in the "Good Challenge" column, do not proceed to the harder client statements but rather repeat the same level.

Making Client Statements Easier

If the therapist ever rates the difficulty of the exercise above an 8 or has any of the reactions in the "Too Hard" column, use the next level easier client statements (e.g., if you were using advanced client statements, switch to intermediate). But if you already were using beginner client statements, use the following methods to make the client statements even easier:

- The person playing the client can use the same beginner client statements but this time in a softer, calmer voice and with a smile. This softens the emotional tone.

FIGURE A.1. Deliberate Practice Reaction Form

Question 1: How challenging was it to fulfill the skill criteria for this exercise?

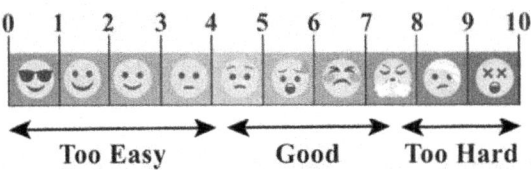

Question 2: Did you have any reactions in "good challenge" or "too hard" categories? (yes/no)					
Good Challenge			**Too Hard**		
Emotions and Thoughts	Body Reactions	Urges	Emotions and Thoughts	Body Reactions	Urges
Manageable shame, self-judgment, irritation, anger, sadness, etc.	Body tension, sighs, shallow breathing, increased heart rate, warmth, dry mouth	Looking away, withdrawing, changing focus	Severe or overwhelming shame, self-judgment, rage, grief, guilt, etc.	Migraines, dizziness, foggy thinking, diarrhea, disassociation, numbness, blanking out, nausea, etc.	Shutting down, giving up

Too Easy ⬇ Proceed to next difficulty level	Good Challenge ⬇ Repeat the same difficulty level	Too Hard ⬇ Go back to previous difficulty level

Note. From *Deliberate Practice in Emotion-Focused Therapy* (p. 180), by R. N. Goldman, A. Vaz, and T. Rousmaniere, 2021, American Psychological Association (https://doi.org/10.1037/0000227-000). Copyright 2021 by the American Psychological Association.

- The client can improvise with topics that are less evocative or make the therapist more comfortable, such as talking about topics without expressing feelings, the future or past (avoiding the here and now), or any topic outside therapy (see Figure A.2).

- The therapist can take a short break (5–10 minutes) between questions.

- The trainer can expand the "feedback phase" by discussing rational emotive behavior therapy or psychotherapy theory and research. This should shift the trainees' focus toward more detached or intellectual topics and reduce the emotional intensity.

Making Client Statements Harder

If the therapist rates the difficulty of the exercise below a 4 or didn't have any of the reactions in the "Good Challenge" column, proceed to next-level, harder client statements. If you were already using the advanced client statements, the client should make the exercise harder, using the following guidelines:

FIGURE A.2. How to Make Client Statements Easier or Harder in Role-Plays

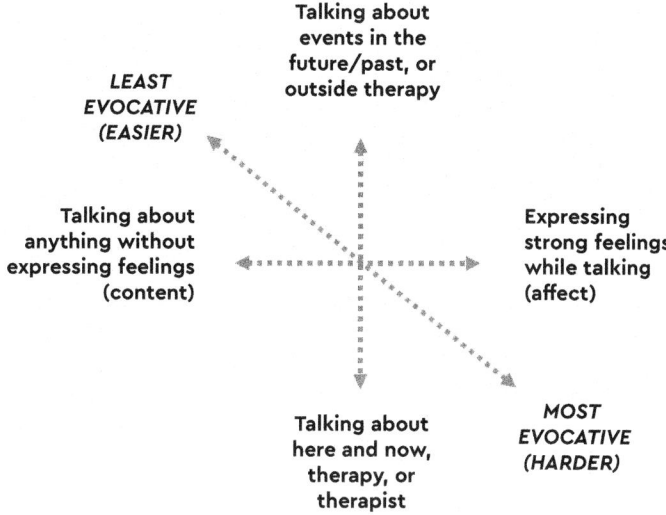

Note. Figure created by Jason Whipple, PhD.

- The person playing the client can use the advanced client statements again with a more distressed voice (e.g., very angry, sad, sarcastic) or unpleasant facial expression. This should increase the emotional tone.

- The client can improvise new client statements with topics that are more evocative or make the therapist uncomfortable, such as expressing strong feelings or talking about the here and now, therapy, or the therapist (see Figure A.2).

Note. The purpose of a deliberate practice session is not to get through all the client statements and therapist responses but to spend as much time as possible practicing at the correct difficulty level. This may mean that trainees repeat the same statements/responses many times, which is okay, as long as the difficulty remains at the "good challenge" level.

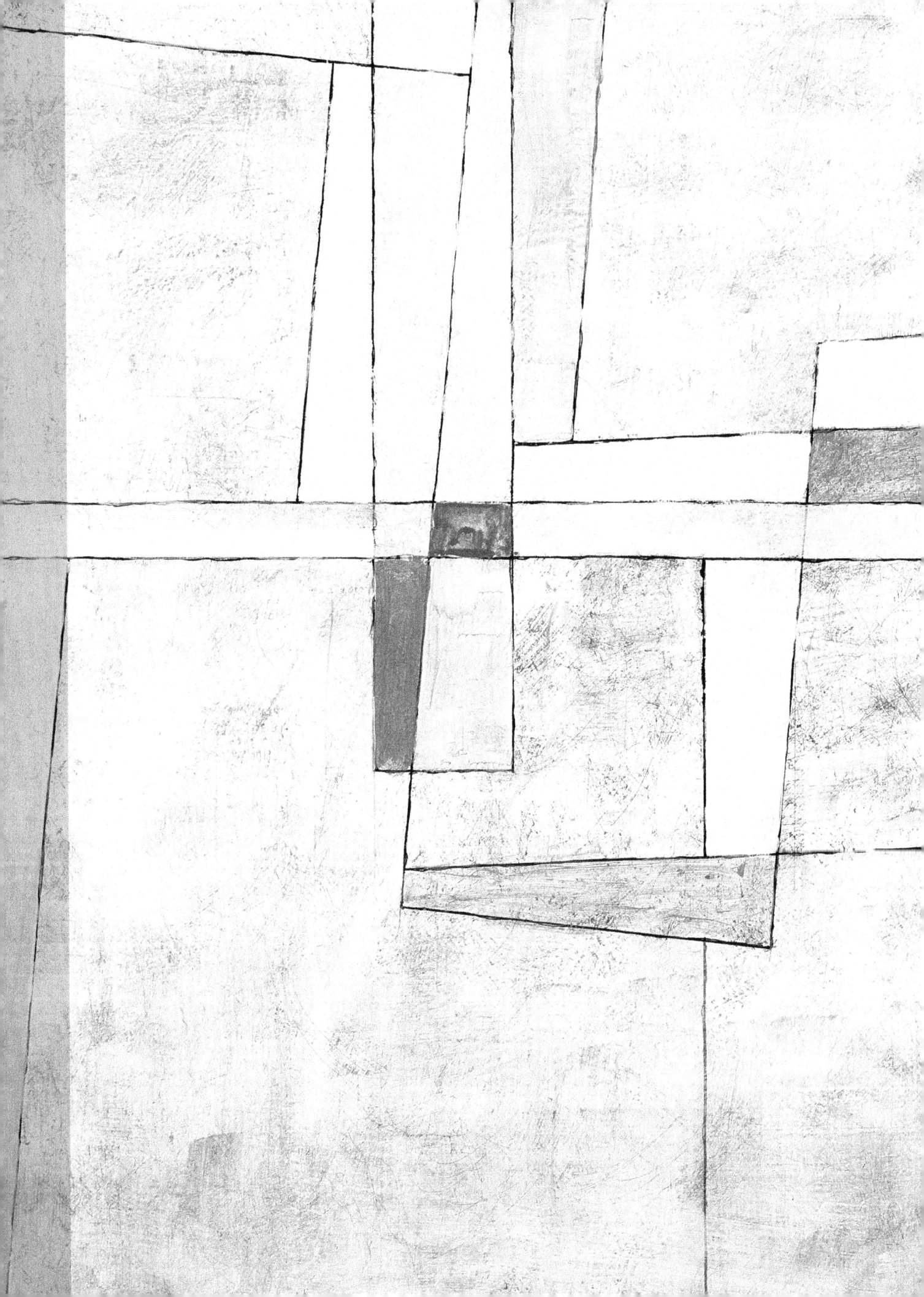

Deliberate Practice Diary Form

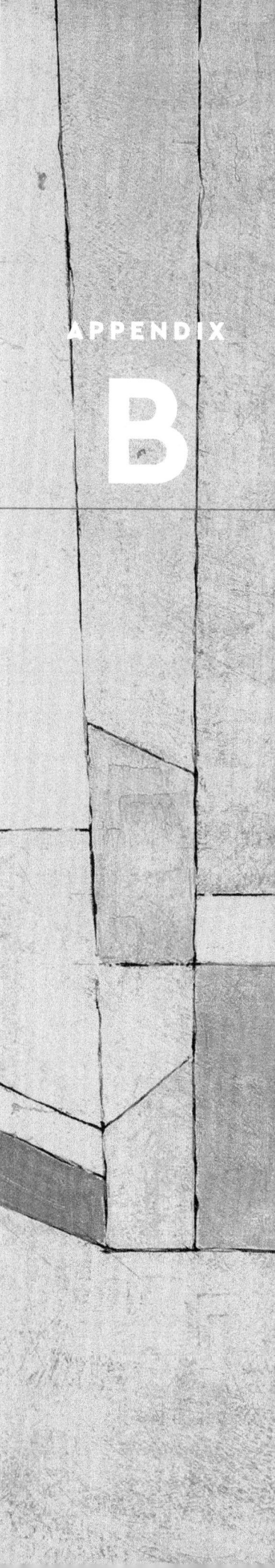

This book focuses on deliberate practice methods that involve active, live engagement between trainees and a supervisor. Importantly, deliberate practice can extend beyond these focused training sessions. For example, a trainee might read the client stimuli quietly or aloud and practice their responses independently between sessions with a supervisor. In such cases, it is important for the trainee to speak aloud rather than rehearse silently in one's head. Alternatively, two trainees can practice without the supervisor. Although the absence of a supervisor limits one source of feedback, the peer trainee who is playing the client can serve this role, as they can when a supervisor is present. Importantly, these additional deliberate practice opportunities are intended to take place between focused training sessions with a supervisor. To optimize the quality of the deliberate practice when conducted independently or without a supervisor, we have developed a Deliberate Practice Diary Form that can also be downloaded from the "Clinician and Practitioner Resources" tab online (https://www.apa.org/pubs/books/deliberate-practice-rational-emotive-behavior-therapy). This form provides a template for the trainee to record their experience of the deliberate practice activity and, ideally, will aid in the consolidation of learning. This form can also be used as part of the evaluation process with the supervisor but is not necessarily intended for that purpose, and trainees are certainly welcome to bring their experience with the independent practice into the next meeting with the supervisor.

Deliberate Practice Diary Form

Use this form to consolidate learnings from the deliberate practice exercises. Please protect your personal boundaries by only sharing information that you are comfortable disclosing.

Name: _____ Date: _____

Exercise: _____

Question 1. What was helpful or worked well this deliberate practice session? In what way?

Question 2. What was unhelpful or didn't go well this deliberate practice session? In what way?

Question 3. What did you learn about yourself, your current skills, and skills you'd like to keep improving? Feel free to share any details, but only those you are comfortable disclosing.

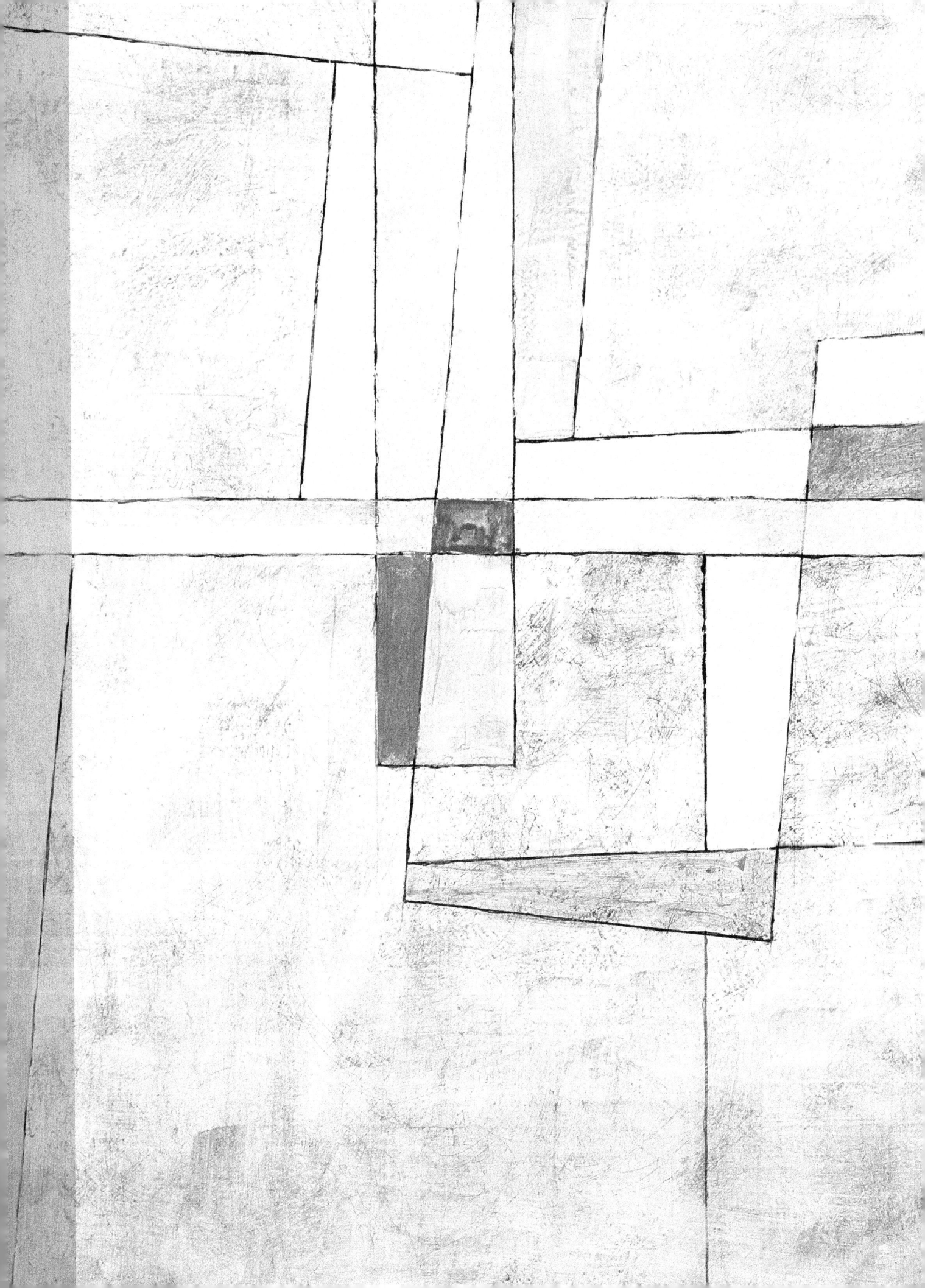

Sample Rational Emotive Behavior Therapy Syllabus With Embedded Deliberate Practice Exercises

This appendix provides a sample one-semester, three-unit course dedicated to teaching rational emotive behavior therapy (REBT). This course is appropriate for graduate students (master's and doctoral students) at all levels of training, including first-year students who have not yet worked with clients. If offering a limited REBT course, aspects of the syllabus and associated exercises can be adapted for use in such a course, in a practicum, in didactic training events at externships and internships, in workshops, and in a continuing education program for postgraduate therapists.

Course Title: Rational Emotive Behavior Therapy: Theory, Clinical Activities, and Deliberate Practice

Course Description

This course teaches beginning practitioners the theory, principles, and core clinical skills of REBT. The course has both didactic and practical elements; it reviews the theory and research on REBT to formulate and understand client problems and employs the deliberate practice approach to guide students to acquire 12 key REBT skills.

Course Objectives

Students who complete this course will be able to

1. Describe the core theory and clinical skills of REBT
2. Apply the principles of deliberate practice for career-long clinical skill development in REBT
3. Demonstrate key REBT skills
4. Evaluate how practitioners can use REBT skills in their work with clients' presenting with several disturbed clinical emotions
5. Employ REBT with clients from a diverse range of cultural backgrounds

Format of Class

Classes are 3 hours long. Course time is split evenly between learning REBT theory (lecture/discussion) and acquiring and practicing REBT skills.

Lecture/Discussion: Each week, class focuses on one lecture/discussion topic for 1.5 hours explaining an aspect of REBT theory and intervention activities.

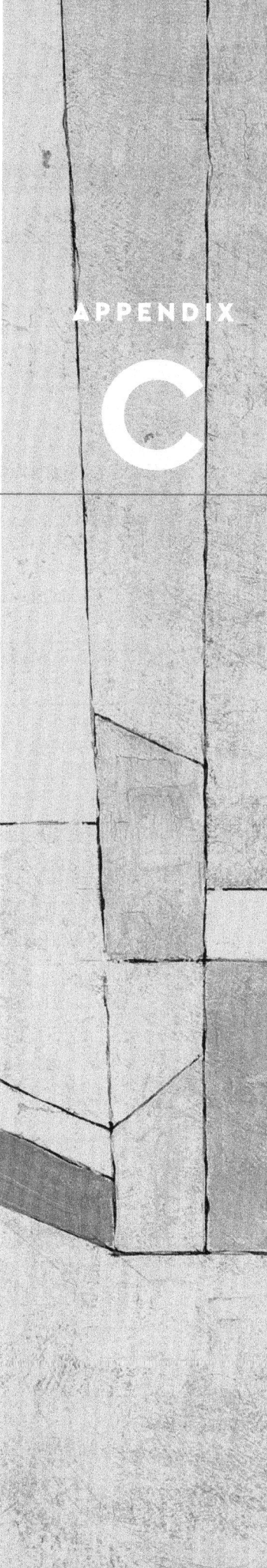

Date	Lecture and Discussion	Skills Lab	Readings
Week 1	Introduction to rational emotive behavior therapy (REBT): history, theory, and research	Exercise 1: Psychoeducation About REBT's ABC Model The ABCs as a case conceptualization model	D. David et al. (2018); O. A. David et al. (2021); DiGiuseppe & Doyle (2019); Hollon & DiGiuseppe (2011); Oltean & David (2018); Vîslă et al. (2016)
Week 2	Basic and current philosophy of REBT, the philosophical foundation of REBT and REBT as a philosophy of life	Exercise 2: Psychoeducation About Dysfunctional Versus Functional Negative Emotions and Behaviors	DiGiuseppe et al. (2014, Chapter 1); A. Ellis (1994); Matweychuk (2022)
Week 3	Common, shared, and unique aspects of REBT; how REBT differs from other forms of cognitive behavior therapy; REBT's place in modern psychotherapy	Exercise 3: Agreement on the Session Goals	DiGiuseppe (2022); DiGiuseppe et al. (2014, Chapter 2); Dryden (2019); Matweychuk et al. (2019)
Week 4	Training in psychotherapy: introduction to principles and advantages of deliberate practice	Exercise 4: Clarifying Inferences From Irrational Beliefs	Rousmaniere (2016); Rousmaniere et al. (2017); Tracey et al. (2014)
Week 5	Teaching clients the ABCs of REBT	Exercise 5: Assessing Irrational Beliefs About the Activating Event	Cristea et al. (2016); DiGiuseppe et al. (2014, Chapter 4); DiGiuseppe and Doyle (2021)
Week 6	Teaching clients about adaptive and maladaptive emotions	Exercise 6: Prioritizing Which Irrational Beliefs to Target for Change	DiGiuseppe et al. (2014, Chapter 8)
Week 7	Establishing the alliance: attaining agreement on the goals of therapy	Exercise 7: Teaching the Belief–Consequence Connection	DiGiuseppe et al. (2014, Chapters 5 & 6); Eubanks et al. (2019)
Week 8	Midterm paper due, self-evaluation, skill feedback	Mock Sessions (beginner profiles)	
Week 9	Distinguishing and assessing beliefs and cognitions	Exercise 8: Functional Disputation of Irrational Beliefs	DiGiuseppe et al. (2014, Chapters 3 & 9)
Week 10	Teaching clients the relationship between beliefs and emotions	Exercise 9: Empirical Disputation of Irrational Beliefs	DiGiuseppe et al. (2014, Chapters 7 & 8)
Week 11	Teaching clients to dispute irrational beliefs	Exercise 10: Semantic Disputation of Irrational Beliefs	DiGiuseppe et al. (2014, Chapters 10, 11, & 13–15); Overholser (2018)
Week 12	Teaching clients to change irrational beliefs; rational replacement beliefs	Exercise 11: Constructing Full Rational Alternative Beliefs to Replace Irrational Beliefs	DiGiuseppe et al. (2014, Chapter 12)
Week 13	Where change happens: the work between sessions	Exercise 12: Collaborative Homework Development	DiGiuseppe et al. (2014, Chapter 16); Kazantzis et al. (2005)
Week 14	Organizing the skills into a whole session	Mock Sessions (intermediate and advanced profiles)	DiGiuseppe et al. (2014, Chapters 17 & 18); Dryden et al. (2010)
Week 15	Final paper due, final exam, self-evaluation, skill feedback	Exam	Annotated therapy transcript

REBT Skills Lab: Each week the students engage in the rehearsal of one REBT skill across several clinical problems typically presented by clients seeking psychotherapy for 1.5 hours. The skills labs primarily focus on practicing REBT skills using the exercises in the REBT deliberate practice book. The exercises use therapy simulations (role-plays) that are designed to accomplish the following goals:

1. Build trainees' skill and confidence for using REBT skills with real client problems
2. Provide students the opportunity to engage in highly structured and repetitive deliberate practice exercises that rehearse the REBT skills
3. Provide a safe space for experimenting with different therapeutic skills and interventions, without fear of criticism for making mistakes
4. Provide opportunities for beginning therapists to explore different styles of therapy so that they can discover their own personal, unique therapy style

Mock Sessions: Twice in the semester (Weeks 8 and 14), trainees will do a psychotherapy mock session in the skills taught in the REBT skills lab. The psychotherapy mock sessions are unstructured role-played therapy sessions. Mock sessions allow trainees to

1. Practice using REBT skills accurately
2. Experiment with clinical decision making concerning which skill to employ in an unscripted context
3. Discover their personal therapeutic style
4. Build self-efficacy for working with real clients

Homework

Homework will be assigned each week and will include reading, 1 hour of skills practice with an assigned practice partner, and occasional writing assignments. For the skills practice homework, trainees will repeat the exercise they did for that week's REBT skills lab. Because the instructor will not be present to evaluate performance, trainees should complete the Deliberate Practice Reaction Form, as well as the Deliberate Practice Diary Form, for themselves as a self-evaluation.

Writing Assignments

Students are to write two papers: one due at midterm and one due on the last day of class. The first paper will explore one aspect of REBT theory or the empirical literature on REBT. The second paper will involve the completion of an REBT case formulation and in accordance with the *Ethical Principles of Psychologists and Code of Conduct* (American Psychological Association, 2017), students are **not required to disclose personal information**. Because this class is about developing both interpersonal and REBT competence, following are some important points so that students are fully informed as they make choices to self-disclose:

- Students choose how much, when, and what to disclose. Students are not penalized for the choice not to share personal information.

- The learning environment is susceptible to group dynamics much like any other group space, and therefore students may be asked to share their observations and experiences of the class environment with the singular goal of fostering a more inclusive and productive learning environment.

Confidentiality

To create a safe learning environment that is respectful of client and therapist information and diversity and to foster open and vulnerable conversation in class, students are
required to agree to strict confidentiality within and outside of the instruction setting.

Evaluation

Self-Evaluation: At the end of the semester (Week 15), trainees will perform a self-evaluation.
This will help trainees track their progress and identify areas for further development. The
"Guidance for Trainees" section in Chapter 3 of *Deliberate Practice in Rational Emotive
Behavior Therapy* highlights potential areas of focus for self-evaluation.

Grading Criteria

Students will be evaluated on the level and quality of their performance in

- the lecture/discussion,
- the skills lab (exercises and mock sessions),
- midterm and final papers, and
- a final exam.

Required Readings

Cristea, I. A., Stefan, S., David, O., Mogoase, C., & Dobrean, A. (2016). *REBT in the treatment
of anxiety disorders in children and adults.* Springer-Nature.

David, D., Cotet, C., Matu, S., Mogoase, C., & Stefan, S. (2018). 50 years of rational-emotive
and cognitive-behavioral therapy: A systematic review and meta-analysis. *Journal of
Clinical Psychology, 74*(3), 304–318. https://doi.org/10.1002/jclp.22514

David, O. A., Cîmpean, A., Costescu, C., DiGiuseppe, R., Doyle, K., Hickey, M., & David, D. (2021).
Effectiveness of outpatient rational emotive behavior therapy. *The American Journal of
Psychotherapy, 74*(4), 157–164. https://doi.org/10.1176/appi.psychotherapy.20200009

DiGiuseppe, R. (2022). REBT's place in modern psychotherapy: Similarities with all psychotherapies, with other forms of CBT, and unique characteristics. In W. Dryden (Ed.), *New
directions in rational emotive behaviour therapy* (pp. 33–54). Routledge/Taylor & Francis.

DiGiuseppe, R., & Doyle, K. (2021). Commentary chapter on "How B-C connection and negotiation of F allow the design and implementation of a cooperative and effective disputing
in rational emotive behavior therapy": REBT's B-C connection and negotiation of F. In
G. M. Ruggiero, G. Caselli, & S. Sassaroli (Eds.), *CBT case formulation as therapeutic process*
(pp. 89–97). Springer-Nature.

DiGiuseppe, R. A., & Doyle, K. A. (2019). Rational emotive behavior therapy. In K. S. Dobson &
D. J. A. Dozois (Eds.), *Handbook of cognitive-behavioral therapies* (4th ed., pp. 191–217).
Guilford Press.

DiGiuseppe, R. A., Doyle, K. A., Dryden, W., & Backx, W. (2014). *A practitioner's guide to rational
emotive behavior therapy* (3rd ed.). Oxford University Press.

Dryden, W. (2019). The distinctive features of rational emotive behavior therapy. In M. E. Bernard
& W. Dryden (Eds.), *Advances in REBT: Theory, practice, research, measurement, prevention
and promotion* (pp. 23–46). Springer-Nature. https://doi.org/10.1007/978-3-319-93118-0_2

Dryden, W., Beal, D., Jones, J., & Trower, P. (2010). The REBT competency scale for clinical and
research applications. *Journal of Rational-Emotive & Cognitive-Behavior Therapy, 28*(4),
165–216. https://doi.org/10.1007/s10942-010-0111-3

Ellis, A. (1994). *Reason and emotion in psychotherapy: A comprehensive method of treating
human disturbances* (Rev. & updated). Carol Publishing Group.

Eubanks, C. F., Muran, J. C., & Safran, J. D. (2019). Repairing alliance ruptures. In J. C. Norcross
& M. J. Lambert (Eds.), *Psychotherapy relationships that work: Evidence-based therapist*

contributions (pp. 549–579). Oxford University Press. https://doi.org/10.1093/med-psych/9780190843953.003.0016

Hollon, S. D., & DiGiuseppe, R. (2011). Cognitive theories of psychotherapy. In J. C. Norcross, G. R. VandenBos, & D. K. Freedheim (Eds.), *History of psychotherapy: Continuity and change* (2nd ed., pp. 203–241). American Psychological Association. https://doi.org/10.1037/12353-007

Kazantzis, N., Lampropoulos, G. K., & Deane, F. P. (2005). A national survey of practicing psychologists' use and attitudes toward homework in psychotherapy. *Journal of Consulting and Clinical Psychology, 73*(4), 742–748. https://doi.org/10.1037/0022-006X.73.4.742

Matweychuk, W., DiGiuseppe, R., & Gulyayeva, O. (2019). A comparison of REBT with other cognitive behavior therapies. In M. E. Bernard & W. Dryden (Eds.), *Advances in REBT: Theory, practice, research, measurement, prevention and promotion* (pp. 47–77). Springer-Nature.

Matweychuk, W. J. (2022). Rational emotive behavior therapy as a philosophy of life. In W. Dryden (Ed.), *New directions in rational emotive behaviour therapy* (pp. 161–180). Routledge/Taylor & Francis.

Oltean, H.-R., & David, D. O. (2018). A meta-analysis of the relationship between rational beliefs and psychological distress. *Journal of Clinical Psychology, 74*(6), 883–895. https://doi.org/10.1002/jclp.22562

Overholser, J. (2018). *The Socratic method of psychotherapy.* Columbia University Press.

Rousmaniere, T. G. (2016). *Deliberate practice for psychotherapists: A guide to improving clinical effectiveness.* Routledge/Taylor & Francis. https://doi.org/10.4324/9781315472256

Rousmaniere, T. G., Goodyear, R., Miller, S. D., & Wampold, B. E. (Eds.). (2017). *The cycle of excellence: Using deliberate practice to improve supervision and training.* John Wiley & Sons. https://doi.org/10.1002/9781119165590

Tracey, T. J. G., Wampold, B. E., Lichtenberg, J. W., & Goodyear, R. K. (2014). Expertise in psychotherapy: An elusive goal? *American Psychologist, 69*(3), 218–229. https://doi.org/10.1037/a0035099

Vîslă, A., Flückiger, C., Grosse Holtforth, M., & David, D. (2016). Irrational beliefs and psychological distress: A meta-analysis. *Psychotherapy and Psychosomatics, 85*(1), 8–15. https://doi.org/10.1159/000441231

Supplemental Readings

Bernard, M. E., & Dryden, W. (Eds.). (2019). *Advances in REBT: Theory, practice, research, measurement, prevention and promotion.* Springer-Nature.

David, D. O., DiGiuseppe, R., Dobrean, A., Păsărelu, C. R., & Balazsi, R. (2019). The measurement of irrationality and rationality. In M. E. Bernard & W. Dryden (Eds.), *Advances in REBT: Theory, practice, research, measurement, prevention and promotion* (pp. 79–100). Springer-Nature.

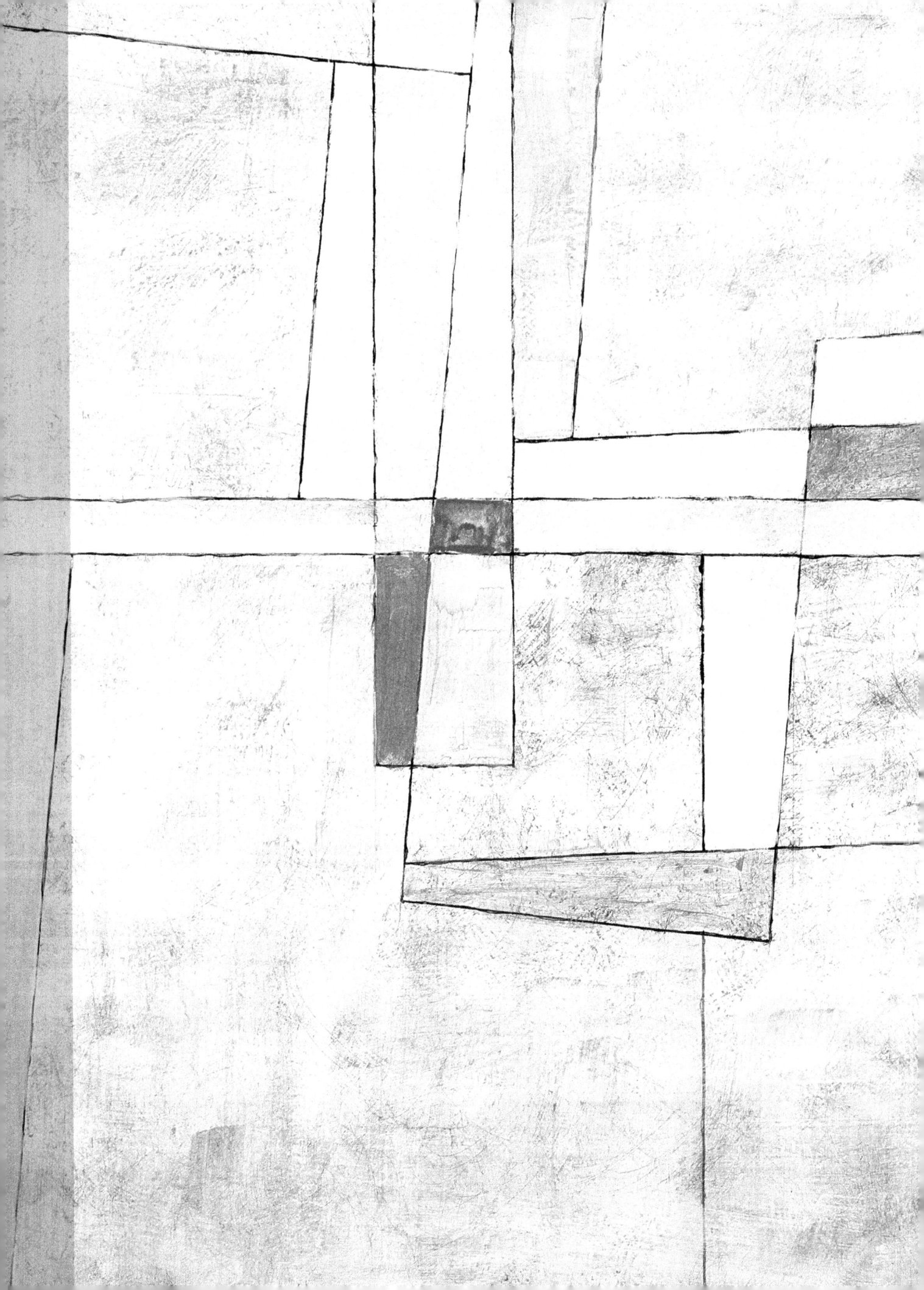

References

American Psychological Association. (2017). *Ethical principles of psychologists and code of conduct.* (2002, amended effective June 1, 2010, and January 1, 2017). https://www.apa.org/ethics/code/

Anderson, T., Ogles, B. M., Patterson, C. L., Lambert, M. J., & Vermeersch, D. A. (2009). Therapist effects: Facilitative interpersonal skills as a predictor of therapist success. *Journal of Clinical Psychology, 65*(7), 755–768. https://doi.org/10.1002/jclp.20583

Bailey, R. J., & Ogles, B. M. (2019, August 1). Common factors as a therapeutic approach: What is required? *Practice Innovations, 4*(4), 241–254. https://doi.org/10.1037/pri0000100

Barlow, D. H. (2010). Negative effects from psychological treatments: A perspective. *American Psychologist, 65*(1), 13–20. https://doi.org/10.1037/a0015643

Bennett-Levy, J. (2019). Why therapists should walk the talk: The theoretical and empirical case for personal practice in therapist training and professional development. *Journal of Behavior Therapy and Experimental Psychiatry, 62,* 133–145. https://doi.org/10.1016/j.jbtep.2018.08.004

Bennett-Levy, J., & Finlay-Jones, A. (2018). The role of personal practice in therapist skill development: A model to guide therapists, educators, supervisors and researchers. *Cognitive Behaviour Therapy, 47*(3), 185–205. https://doi.org/10.1080/16506073.2018.1434678

Bohart, A. C., & Wade, A. G. (2013). The client in psychotherapy. In M. J. Lambert (Ed.), *Bergin and Garfield's handbook of psychotherapy and behavior change* (6th ed., 219–257). John Wiley & Sons.

Bugatti, M., & Boswell, J. F. (2016). Clinical errors as a lack of context responsiveness. *Psychotherapy: Theory, Research, & Practice, 53*(3), 262–267. https://doi.org/10.1037/pst0000080

Carter, L. A., & Barnett, J. E. (2014). *Self-care for clinicians in training: A guide to psychological wellness for graduate students in psychology.* Oxford University Press.

Caspar, F., Berger, T., & Hautle, I. (2004). The right view of your patient: A computer-assisted, individualized module for psychotherapy training. *Psychotherapy: Theory, Research, & Practice, 41*(2), 125–135. https://doi.org/10.1037/0033-3204.41.2.125

Castonguay, L. G., Goldfried, M. R., Wiser, S., Raue, P. J., & Hayes, A. M. (1996). Predicting the effect of cognitive therapy for depression: A study of unique and common factors. *Journal of Consulting and Clinical Psychology, 64*(3), 497–504. https://doi.org/10.1037/0022-006X.64.3.497

Chow, D. L., Miller, S. D., Seidel, J. A., Kane, R. T., Thornton, J. A., & Andrews, W. P. (2015). The role of deliberate practice in the development of highly effective psychotherapists. *Psychotherapy: Theory, Research, & Practice, 52*(3), 337–345. https://doi.org/10.1037/pst0000015

Coker, J. (1990). *How to practice jazz.* Jamey Aebersold.

Cook, R. (2005). *It's about that time: Miles Davis on and off record.* Atlantic Books.

Coughlan, E. K., Williams, A. M., McRobert, A. P., & Ford, P. R. (2014). How experts practice: A novel test of deliberate practice theory. *Journal of Experimental Psychology: Learning, Memory, and Cognition, 40*(2), 449–458. https://doi.org/10.1037/a0034302

Cristea, I. A., Stefan, S., David, O., Mogoase, C., & Dobrean, A. (2016). *REBT in the treatment of anxiety disorders in children and adults.* Springer-Nature.

Csikszentmihalyi, M. (1997). *Finding flow: The psychology of engagement with everyday life.* Harper Collins.

David, D., Cotet, C., Matu, S., Mogoase, C., & Stefan, S. (2018). 50 years of rational-emotive and cognitive-behavioral therapy: A systematic review and meta-analysis. *Journal of Clinical Psychology, 74*(3), 304–318. https://doi.org/10.1002/jclp.22514

David, O. A., Cîmpean, A., Costescu, C., DiGiuseppe, R., Doyle, K., Hickey, M., & David, D. (2021). Effectiveness of outpatient rational emotive behavior therapy. *The American Journal of Psychotherapy, 74*(4), 157–164. https://doi.org/10.1176/appi.psychotherapy.20200009

Davis, D. E., DeBlaere, C., Owen, J., Hook, J. N., Rivera, D. P., Choe, E., Van Tongeren, D. R., Worthington, E. L., & Placeres, V. (2018). The multicultural orientation framework: A narrative review. *Psychotherapy: Theory, Research, & Practice, 55*(1), 89–100. https://doi.org/10.1037/pst0000160

DiGiuseppe, R. (2022). REBT's place in modern psychotherapy: Similarities with all psychotherapies, with other forms of CBT, and unique characteristics. In W. Dryden (Ed.), *New directions in rational emotive behaviour therapy* (pp. 33–54). Routledge/Taylor & Francis.

DiGiuseppe, R., & Doyle, K. (2021). Commentary chapter on "How B-C connection and negotiation of F allow the design and implementation of a cooperative and effective disputing in rational emotive behavior therapy": REBT's B-C connection and negotiation of F. In G. M. Ruggiero, G. Caselli, & S. Sassaroli (Eds.), *CBT case formulation as therapeutic process* (pp. 89–97). Springer-Nature.

DiGiuseppe, R., Gorman, B., & Raptis, J. (2020). The Factor Structure of the Attitudes and Beliefs Scale 2: Implications for rational emotive behavior therapy. *Journal of Rational-Emotive & Cognitive-Behavior Therapy, 38*(2), 111–142. https://doi.org/10.1007/s10942-020-00349-0

DiGiuseppe, R. A., & Doyle, K. A. (2019). Rational emotive behavior therapy. In K. S. Dobson & D. J. A. Dozois (Eds.), *Handbook of cognitive-behavioral therapies* (4th ed., pp. 191–217). Guilford Press.

DiGiuseppe, R. A., Doyle, K. A., Dryden, W., & Backx, W. (2014). *A practitioner's guide to rational emotive behavior therapy* (3rd ed.). Oxford University Press.

Doyle, K., Hickey, M., & DiGiuseppe, R. (2022). Supervision in rational emotive behavior therapy. In C. A. Storch, J. S. Abramowitz, & D. McKay (Eds.), *Training and supervision in specialized cognitive-behavior therapy: Methods, settings, & populations* (pp. 37–49). American Psychological Association. https://doi.org/10.1037/0000314-004

Dryden, W. (2001). *Reason to change: A rational emotive behaviour therapy (REBT) workbook.* Brunner/Routledge.

Dryden, W. (2019). The distinctive features of rational emotive behavior therapy. In M. E. Bernard & W. Dryden (Eds.), *Advances in REBT: Theory, practice, research, measurement, prevention and promotion* (pp. 23–46). Springer-Nature. https://doi.org/10.1007/978-3-319-93118-0_2

Dryden, W. (2020). Awfulizing: Some conceptual and therapeutic considerations. *Journal of Rational-Emotive & Cognitive-Behavior Therapy, 38*(3), 295–305. https://doi.org/10.1007/s10942-020-00358-z

Dryden, W., Beal, D., Jones, J., & Trower, P. (2010). The REBT competency scale for clinical and research applications. *Journal of Rational-Emotive & Cognitive-Behavior Therapy, 28*(4), 165–216. https://doi.org/10.1007/s10942-010-0111-3

Dryden, W., David, D., & Ellis, A. (2010). Rational emotive behavior therapy. In K. S. Dobson (Ed.), *Handbook of cognitive-behavioral therapies* (3rd ed., pp. 226–276). Guilford Press.

Ellis, A. (1957). Rational psychotherapy and individual psychology. *Journal of Individual Psychology, 13*, 38–44.

Ellis, A. (1962). *Reason and emotion in psychotherapy*. Lyle Stuart.

Ellis, A. (1994). *Reason and emotion in psychotherapy: A comprehensive method of treating human disturbances* (Rev. & updated). Carol Publishing Group.

Ellis, M. V., Berger, L., Hanus, A. E., Ayala, E. E., Swords, B. A., & Siembor, M. (2014). Inadequate and harmful clinical supervision: Testing a revised framework and assessing occurrence. *The Counseling Psychologist, 42*(4), 434–472. https://doi.org/10.1177/0011000013508656

Ericsson, K. A. (2003). Development of elite performance and deliberate practice: An update from the perspective of the expert performance approach. In J. L. Starkes & K. A. Ericsson (Eds.), *Expert performance in sports: Advances in research on sport expertise* (pp. 49–83). Human Kinetics.

Ericsson, K. A. (2004). Deliberate practice and the acquisition and maintenance in medicine and related domains: Invited address. *Academic Medicine, 79*, S70–S81. https://doi.org/10.1097/00001888-200410001-00022

Ericsson, K. A. (2006). The influence of experience and deliberate practice on the development of superior expert performance. In K. A. Ericsson, N. Charness, P. J. Feltovich, & R. R. Hoffman (Eds.), *The Cambridge handbook of expertise and expert performance* (pp. 683–703). Cambridge University Press. https://doi.org/10.1017/CBO9780511816796.038

Ericsson, K. A., Hoffman, R. R., Kozbelt, A., & Williams, A. M. (Eds.). (2018). *The Cambridge handbook of expertise and expert performance* (2nd ed.). Cambridge University Press. https://doi.org/10.1017/9781316480748

Ericsson, K. A., Krampe, R. T., & Tesch-Römer, C. (1993). The role of deliberate practice in the acquisition of expert performance. *Psychological Review, 100*(3), 363–406. https://doi.org/10.1037/0033-295X.100.3.363

Ericsson, K. A., & Pool, R. (2016). *Peak: Secrets from the new science of expertise*. Houghton Mifflin Harcourt.

Eubanks, C. F., Muran, J. C., & Safran, J. D. (2019). Repairing alliance ruptures. In J. C. Norcross & M. J. Lambert (Eds.), *Psychotherapy relationships that work: Evidence-based therapist contributions* (pp. 549–579). Oxford University Press. https://doi.org/10.1093/med-psych/9780190843953.003.0016

Eubanks-Carter, C., Muran, J. C., & Safran, J. D. (2015). Alliance-focused training. *Psychotherapy, 52*(2), 169–173. https://doi.org/10.1037/a0037596

Fisher, R. P., & Craik, F. I. (1977). Interaction between encoding and retrieval operations in cued recall. *Journal of Experimental Psychology: Human Learning and Memory, 3*(6), 701–711. https://doi.org/10.1037/0278-7393.3.6.701

Fouad, N. A., Hatcher, R. L., Hutchings, P. S., Collins, F. L., Grus, C. L., Kaslow, N. J., Madson, M. B., & Crossman, R. E. (2009). Competency benchmarks: A model for understanding and measuring competence in professional psychology across training levels. *Training and Education in Professional Psychology, 3*(4, Suppl.), S5–S26. https://doi.org/10.1037/a0015832

Gladwell, M. (2008). *Outliers: The story of success*. Little, Brown & Company.

Goldberg, S., Rousmaniere, T. G., Miller, S. D., Whipple, J., Nielsen, S. L., Hoyt, W., & Wampold, B. E. (2016). Do psychotherapists improve with time and experience? A longitudinal analysis of outcomes in a clinical setting. *Journal of Counseling Psychology, 63*, 1–11. https://doi.org/10.1037/cou0000131

Goldberg, S. B., Babins-Wagner, R., Rousmaniere, T., Berzins, S., Hoyt, W. T., Whipple, J. L., Miller, S. D., & Wampold, B. E. (2016). Creating a climate for therapist improvement: A case study of an agency focused on outcomes and deliberate practice. *Psychotherapy: Theory, Research, & Practice, 53*(3), 367–375. https://doi.org/10.1037/pst0000060

Goldman, R. N., Vaz, A., & Rousmaniere, T. (2021). *Deliberate practice in emotion-focused therapy*. American Psychological Association. https://doi.org/10.1037/0000227-000

Goodyear, R. K. (2015). Using accountability mechanisms more intentionally: A framework and its implications for training professional psychologists. *American Psychologist, 70*(8), 736–743. https://doi.org/10.1037/a0039828

Goodyear, R. K., & Nelson, M. L. (1997). The major formats of psychotherapy supervision. In C. E. Watkins, Jr. (Ed.), *Handbook of psychotherapy supervision* (pp. 328–344). John Wiley & Sons.

Goodyear, R. K., & Rousmaniere, T. G. (2017). Helping therapists to each day become a little better than they were the day before: The expertise-development model of supervision and consultation. In T. G. Rousmaniere, R. Goodyear, S. D. Miller, & B. Wampold (Eds.), *The cycle of excellence: Using deliberate practice to improve supervision and training* (pp. 67–95). John Wiley & Sons. https://doi.org/10.1002/9781119165590.ch4

Goodyear, R. K., Wampold, B. E., Tracey, T. J. G., & Lichtenberg, J. W. (2017). Psychotherapy expertise should mean superior outcomes and demonstrable improvement over time. *The Counseling Psychologist, 45*(1), 54–65. https://doi.org/10.1177/0011000016652691

Hackney, H. L., & Bernard, J. M. (2017). *Professional counseling: A process guide to helping* (8th ed.). Pearson.

Haggerty, G., & Hilsenroth, M. J. (2011). The use of video in psychotherapy supervision. *British Journal of Psychotherapy, 27*(2), 193–210. https://doi.org/10.1111/j.1752-0118.2011.01232.x

Harris, J., Jin, J., Hoffman, S., Phan, S., Prout, T. A., Rousmaniere, T., & Vaz, A. (in press). *Deliberate practice in multicultural therapy.* American Psychological Association.

Hatcher, R. L. (2015). Interpersonal competencies: Responsiveness, technique, and training in psychotherapy. *American Psychologist, 70*(8), 747–757. https://doi.org/10.1037/a0039803

Hayes, S. C., Follette, V. M., & Linehan, M. M. (Eds.). (2004). *Mindfulness and acceptance: Expanding the cognitive behavioral tradition.* Guilford Press.

Hembree, E. A., Rauch, S. A. M., & Foa, E. B. (2003). Beyond the manual: The insider's guide to prolonged exposure therapy for PTSD. *Cognitive and Behavioral Practice, 10*(1), 22–30. https://doi.org/10.1016/S1077-7229(03)80005-6

Henry, W. P., Strupp, H. H., Butler, S. F., Schacht, T. E., & Binder, J. L. (1993). Effects of training in time-limited dynamic psychotherapy: Changes in therapist behavior. *Journal of Consulting and Clinical Psychology, 61*(3), 434–440. https://doi.org/10.1037/0022-006X.61.3.434

Hill, C. E., Kivlighan, D. M., III, Rousmaniere, T., Kivlighan, D. M., Jr., Gerstenblith, J. A., & Hillman, J. W. (2020). Deliberate practice for the skill of immediacy: A multiple case study of doctoral student therapists and clients. *Psychotherapy, 57*(4), 587–597. https://doi.org/10.1037/pst0000247

Hill, C. E., & Knox, S. (2013). Training and supervision in psychotherapy: Evidence for effective practice. In M. J. Lambert (Ed.), *Handbook of psychotherapy and behavior change* (6th ed., pp. 775–811). Wiley.

Hollon, S. D., & DiGiuseppe, R. (2011). Cognitive theories of psychotherapy. In J. C. Norcross, G. R. VandenBos, & D. K. Freedheim (Eds.), *History of psychotherapy: Continuity and change* (2nd ed., pp. 203–241). American Psychological Association. https://doi.org/10.1037/12353-007

Hook, J. N., Davis, D. D., Owen, J., & DeBlaere, C. (2017). *Cultural humility: Engaging diverse identities in therapy.* American Psychological Association. https://doi.org/10.1037/0000037-000

Kaslow, N. J., Campbell, L. F., Hatcher, R. L., Grus, C. L., Fouad, N. A., & Rodolfa, E. R. (2009). Competency assessment toolkit for professional psychology. *Training and Education in Professional Psychology, 3*(4, Suppl.), S27–S45. https://doi.org/10.1037/a0015833

Kazantzis, N., Lampropoulos, G. K., & Deane, F. P. (2005). A national survey of practicing psychologists' use and attitudes toward homework in psychotherapy. *Journal of Consulting and Clinical Psychology, 73*(4), 742–748. https://doi.org/10.1037/0022-006X.73.4.742

Kendall, P. C., & Beidas, R. S. (2007). Smoothing the trail for dissemination of evidence-based practices for youth: Flexibility within fidelity. *Professional Psychology, Research and Practice, 38*(1), 13–19. https://doi.org/10.1037/0735-7028.38.1.13

Kendall, P. C., & Frank, H. E. (2018). Implementing evidence-based treatment protocols: Flexibility within fidelity. *Clinical Psychology: Science and Practice, 25*(4), e12271. https://doi.org/10.1111/cpsp.12271

Koziol, L. F., & Budding, D. E. (2012). Procedural learning. In N. M. Seel (Ed.), *Encyclopedia of the science of learning* (pp. 2694–2696). Springer. https://doi.org/10.1007/978-1-4419-1428-6_670

Lambert, M. J. (2010). Yes, it is time for clinicians to monitor treatment outcome. In B. L. Duncan, S. C. Miller, B. E. Wampold, & M. A. Hubble (Eds.), *Heart and soul of change:*

Delivering what works in therapy (2nd ed., pp. 239–266). American Psychological Association. https://doi.org/10.1037/12075-008

Markman, K. D., & Tetlock, P. E. (2000). Accountability and close-call counterfactuals: The loser who nearly won and the winner who nearly lost. *Personality and Social Psychology Bulletin, 26*(10), 1213–1224. https://doi.org/10.1177/0146167200262004

Martin, D. (2015). *Counseling skills and therapy* (2nd ed.). Brooks/Cole.

Matweychuk, W., DiGiuseppe, R., & Gulyayeva, O. (2019). A comparison of REBT with other cognitive behavior therapies. In M. E. Bernard & W. Dryden (Eds.), *Advances in REBT: Theory, practice, research, measurement, prevention and promotion* (pp. 47–77). Springer-Nature.

Matweychuk, W. J. (2022). Rational emotive behavior therapy as a philosophy of life. In W. Dryden (Ed.), *New directions in rational emotive behaviour therapy* (pp. 161–180). Routledge/Taylor & Francis.

McGaghie, W. C., Issenberg, S. B., Barsuk, J. H., & Wayne, D. B. (2014). A critical review of simulation-based mastery learning with translational outcomes. *Medical Education, 48*(4), 375–385. https://doi.org/10.1111/medu.12391

McLeod, J. (2017). Qualitative methods for routine outcome measurement. In T. G. Rousmaniere, R. Goodyear, D. D. Miller, & B. E. Wampold (Eds.), *The cycle of excellence: Using deliberate practice to improve supervision and training* (pp. 99–122). John Wiley & Sons. https://doi.org/10.1002/9781119165590.ch5

Muran, J. C., Safran, J. D., & Eubanks-Carter, C. (2010). Developing therapist abilities to negotiate alliance ruptures. In J. C. Muran & J. P. Barber (Eds.), *The therapeutic alliance: An evidence-based guide to practice* (pp. 320–340). Guilford Press.

Norcross, J. C., & Guy, J. D. (2005). The prevalence and parameters of personal therapy in the United States. In J. D. Geller, J. C. Norcross, & D. E. Orlinsky (Eds.), *The psychotherapist's own psychotherapy: Patient and clinician perspectives* (pp. 165–176). Oxford University Press.

Norcross, J. C., Lambert, M. J., & Wampold, B. E. (2019). *Psychotherapy relationships that work* (3rd ed.). Oxford University Press.

Oltean, H.-R., & David, D. O. (2018). A meta-analysis of the relationship between rational beliefs and psychological distress. *Journal of Clinical Psychology, 74*(6), 883–895. https://doi.org/10.1002/jclp.22562

Orlinsky, D. E., & Ronnestad, M. H. (2005). *How psychotherapists develop.* American Psychological Association.

Overholser, J. (2018). *The Socratic method of psychotherapy.* Columbia University Press.

Owen, J., & Hilsenroth, M. J. (2014). Treatment adherence: The importance of therapist flexibility in relation to therapy outcomes. *Journal of Counseling Psychology, 61*(2), 280–288. https://doi.org/10.1037/a0035753

Prescott, D. S., Maeschalck, C. L., & Miller, S. D. (Eds.). (2017). *Feedback-informed treatment in clinical practice: Reaching for excellence.* American Psychological Association. https://doi.org/10.1037/0000039-000

Rousmaniere, T. G. (2016). *Deliberate practice for psychotherapists: A guide to improving clinical effectiveness.* Routledge/Taylor & Francis. https://doi.org/10.4324/9781315472256

Rousmaniere, T. G. (2019). *Mastering the inner skills of psychotherapy: A deliberate practice handbook.* Gold Lantern Press.

Rousmaniere, T. G., Goodyear, R., Miller, S. D., & Wampold, B. E. (Eds.). (2017). *The cycle of excellence: Using deliberate practice to improve supervision and training.* John Wiley & Sons. https://doi.org/10.1002/9781119165590

Squire, L. R. (2004). Memory systems of the brain: A brief history and current perspective. *Neurobiology of Learning and Memory, 82*(3), 171–177. https://doi.org/10.1016/j.nlm.2004.06.005

Stiles, W. B., Honos Webb, L., & Surko, M. (1998). Responsiveness in psychotherapy. *Clinical Psychology: Science and Practice, 5*(4), 439–458. https://doi.org/10.1111/j.1468-2850.1998.tb00166.x

Stiles, W. B., & Horvath, A. O. (2017). Appropriate responsiveness as a contribution to therapist effects. In L. G. Castonguay & C. E. Hill (Eds.), *How and why are some therapists better* than others? *Understanding therapist effects* (pp. 71–84). American Psychological Association. https://doi.org/10.1037/0000034-005

Taylor, J. M., & Neimeyer, G. J. (2017). The ongoing evolution of continuing education: Past, present, and future. In T. G. Rousmaniere, R. Goodyear, S. D. Miller, & B. Wampold (Eds.), *The cycle of excellence: Using deliberate practice to improve supervision and training* (pp. 219–248). John Wiley & Sons.

Tracey, T. J. G., Wampold, B. E., Goodyear, R. K., & Lichtenberg, J. W. (2015). Improving expertise in psychotherapy. *Psychotherapy Bulletin, 50*(1), 7–13.

Tracey, T. J. G., Wampold, B. E., Lichtenberg, J. W., & Goodyear, R. K. (2014). Expertise in psychotherapy: An elusive goal? *American Psychologist, 69*(3), 218–229. https://doi.org/10.1037/a0035099

Turner, M. J. (2016). Rational emotive behavior therapy (REBT), irrational and rational beliefs, and the mental health of athletes. *Frontiers in Psychology, 7*, 1423. https://doi.org/10.3389/fpsyg.2016.01423

Vîslă, A., Flückiger, C., Grosse Holtforth, M., & David, D. (2016). Irrational beliefs and psychological distress: A meta-analysis. *Psychotherapy and Psychosomatics, 85*(1), 8–15. https://doi.org/10.1159/000441231

Wampold, B. E., & Imel, Z. E. (2015). *The great psychotherapy debate: The evidence for what makes psychotherapy work* (2nd ed.). Routledge. https://doi.org/10.4324/9780203582015

Wass, R., & Golding, C. (2014). Sharpening a tool for teaching: The zone of proximal development. *Teaching in Higher Education, 19*(6), 671–684. https://doi.org/10.1080/13562517.2014.901958

Zaretskii, V. (2009). The zone of proximal development: What Vygotsky did not have time to write. *Journal of Russian & East European Psychology, 47*(6), 70–93. https://doi.org/10.2753/RPO1061-0405470604

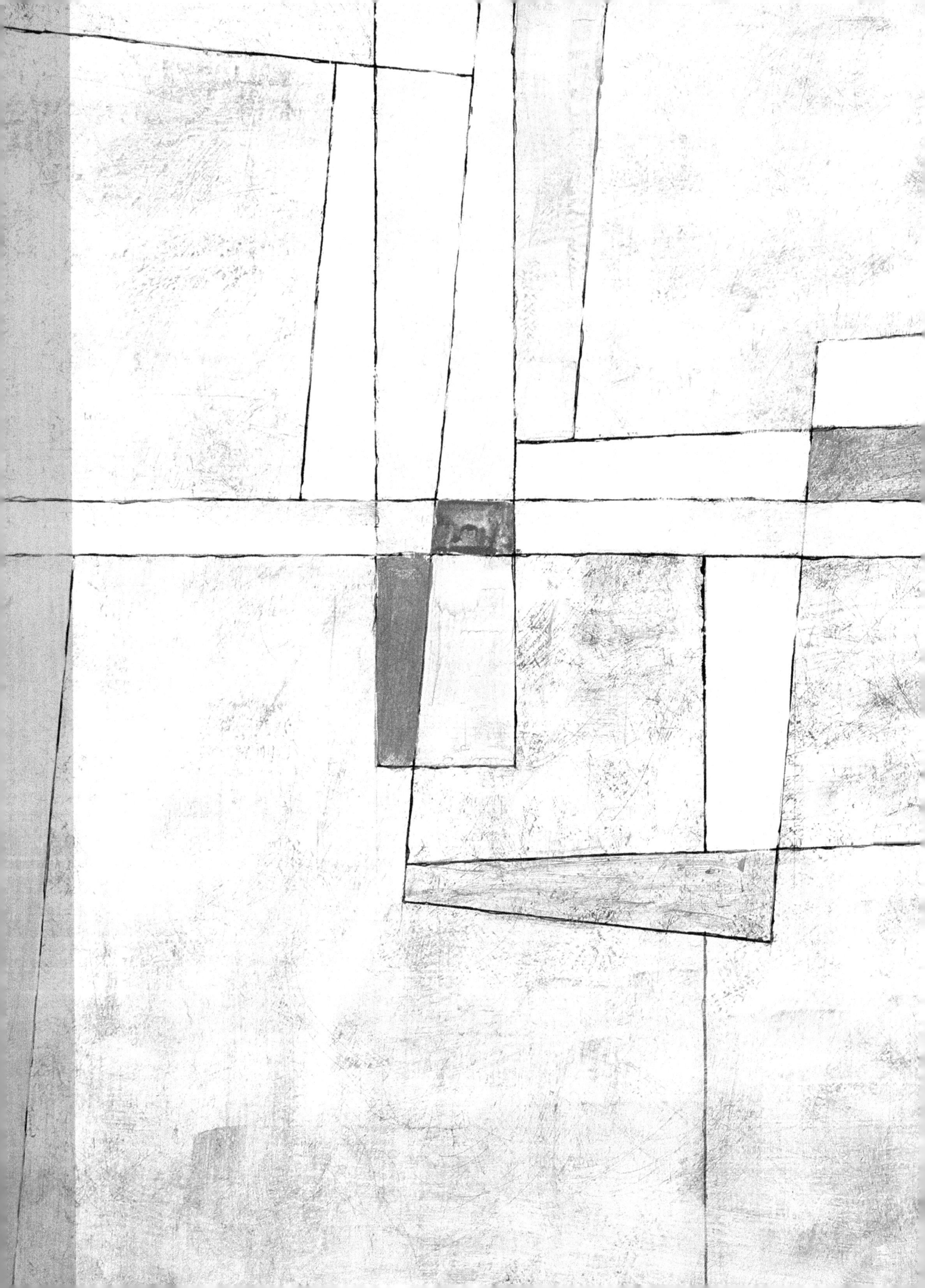

Index

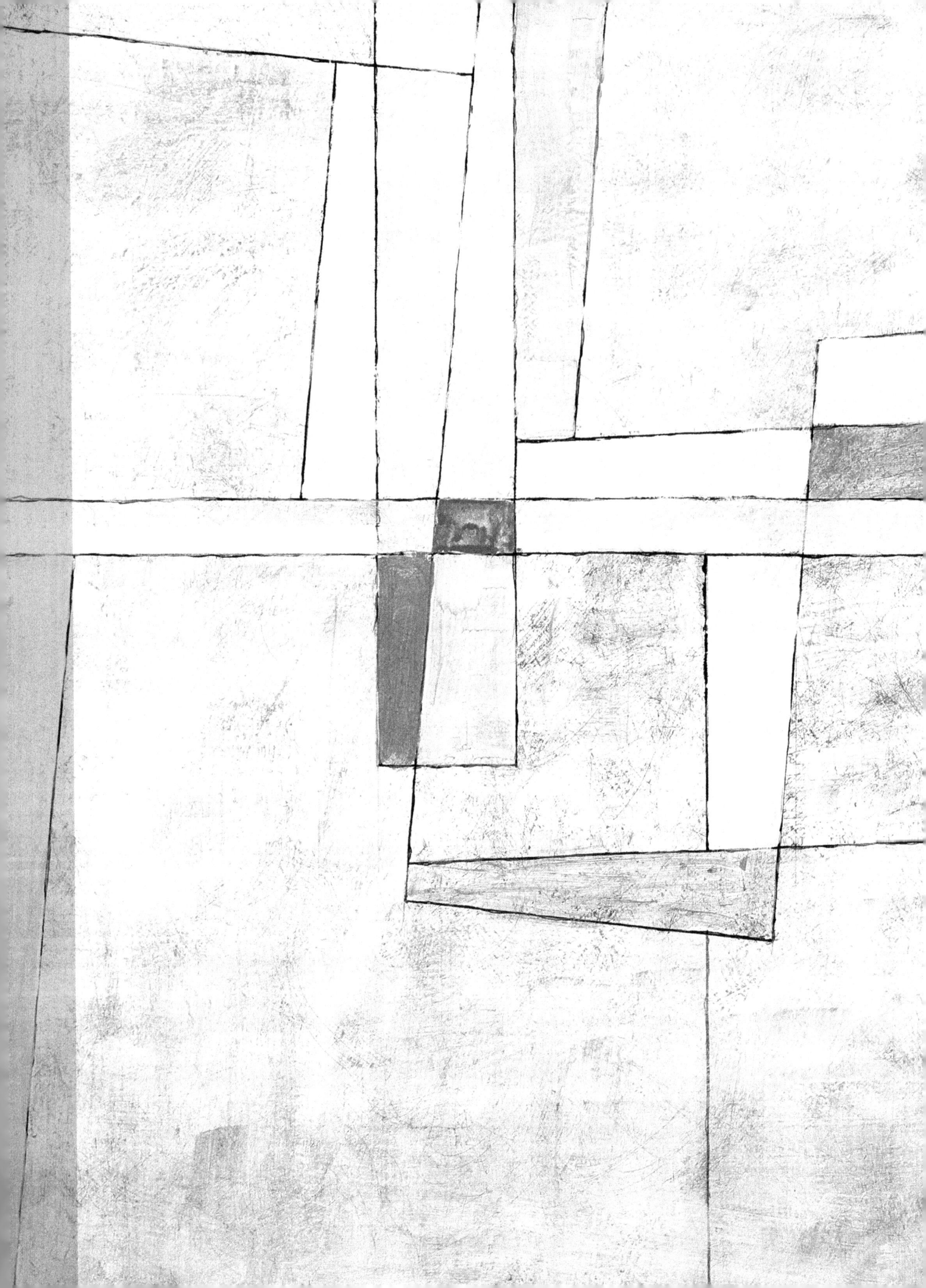

About the Authors

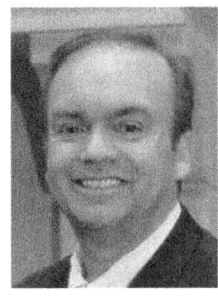

Mark D. Terjesen, PhD, is a professor of psychology and assistant chairperson in the Department of Psychology at St. John's University in Queens, New York. He has served as program director of the School Psychology (PsyD and MS) programs and has trained and supervised doctoral students throughout his tenure, having mentored more than 100 doctoral dissertation research projects. Dr. Terjesen has studied, published, and presented at a number of national and international conferences on topics related to assessment and clinical work with children, adolescents, and families. He has trained many professionals internationally in the use of rational emotive behavior therapy (REBT) and cognitive behavioral practices. Dr. Terjesen has served as president of the School Division of the New York State Psychological Association, president of the Trainers of School Psychologists, and is past president of Division 52 (International Psychology) of the American Psychological Association, of which he is also a fellow. Dr. Terjesen is a fellow of the Albert Ellis Institute and an approved supervisor. He serves as the clinical director at North Coast Psychological Services in Syosset, New York. Dr. Terjesen and his wife, Dr. Carolyn Waldecker, are the proud parents of Amelia Grace, who has taught them how to apply the principles of REBT in their role as parents.

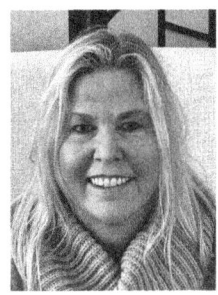

Kristene A. Doyle, PhD, ScD, is the director of the Albert Ellis Institute (AEI). She is also director of clinical services, founding director of the Eating Disorders Treatment and Research Center, and a licensed psychologist at AEI. During her 22-year tenure at AEI, Dr. Doyle has held various leadership roles, including associate executive director, training and development coordinator, and director of child and family services. She is also a diplomate in rational emotive behavior therapy (REBT) and serves on the Diplomate Board. In addition to training and supervising AEI's fellows and staff therapists, Dr. Doyle conducts numerous workshops and professional trainings throughout the world. With a distinguished international presence, she has influenced the growth and practice of REBT in countries spanning several continents, including North America, South America, Europe, Asia, and Africa. Dr. Doyle's clinical and research interests include eating disorders and weight management, REBT treatment of children and adolescents, and the cognitive behavioral therapeutic process, outcome, and dissemination. Dr. Doyle is coauthor of *A Practitioner's Guide to Rational Emotive Behavior Therapy* (3rd ed.). She is also the coeditor of *Cognitive Behavior Therapies: A Guidebook for Practitioners* and of the *Journal of Rational-Emotive & Cognitive-Behavior Therapy*. She has contributed numerous book chapters on topics such as the treatment of eating disorders, attention-deficit/hyperactivity disorder, group therapy, and coping with loss. She has presented her research at several national and international conventions, including those of the American Psychological Association, Association for Behavioral and Cognitive Therapies, and the World Congress of Behavioral and Cognitive Therapies. In addition, Dr. Doyle has published in numerous scientific journals, some of which include *Social Behavior and Personality: An International Journal* and the *Journal of Rational-Emotive & Cognitive-Behavior Therapy*. In addition to her work at AEI, Dr. Doyle is appointed as full adjunct professor at St. John's University in both the Clinical Psychology and School Psychology Doctoral Programs, where she has taught for 22 years, as well as Teachers College, Columbia University.

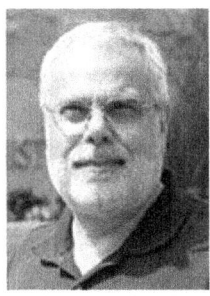

Raymond A. DiGiuseppe, PhD, ScD, earned a BS degree from Villanova University and received his PhD from Hofstra University in 1975. He completed a postdoctoral fellowship at the Albert Ellis Institute (AEI) in 1977. In 1980, he became the institute's director of professional education, a position he has held since. He is also a core faculty trainer for AEI. He has trained hundreds of therapists in rational emotive behavior therapy (REBT) and lectured to thousands throughout the world. He received the Jack D. Krasner Early Career Contribution Award from the American Psychological Association's (APA's) Division 29 (Society for the Advancement of Psychotherapy) and was elected a Fellow of the APA's divisions of Psychotherapy, Clinical, School, and Family Psychology.

Dr. DiGiuseppe joined the faculty of St. John's University in 1987 and is currently a professor of psychology. He has been active in the Association for Behavioral and Cognitive Therapies (ABCT). He helped develop the Diplomate in Behavioral Psychology (1986 1987) and served on the Diplomate board. He was ABCT's associate program chair (1995) and program chair (1996). He has served on the editorial board of ABCT's *Cognitive and Behavioral Practice*. Dr. DiGiuseppe served as ABCT convention coordinator (1997–2000) and associate convener for the 2001 World Congress for Behavior Therapy. He developed popular convention formats such as the Master Clinician Series and the World Rounds demonstrations. He was elected ABCT representative-at-large in 2001 and served as president of the organization in 2006–2007. Dr. DiGiuseppe has also been active in the Society for the Advancement of Psychotherapy (APA Division 29). He served on their Publication Board and was elected president in 2014. He currently serves on the editorial board of the society's journal, *Psychotherapy*.

Dr. DiGiuseppe has contributed to the scientific and clinical literature with six books, more than 150 chapters and articles, and hundreds of conference presentations. He coauthored two psychological tests: the Anger Disorders Scale (for adults) and the Anger Regulation and Expression Scale (for children and adolescents). He coauthored several books on REBT, including *The Practitioner's Guide to Rational Emotive Behavior Therapy*, which is in its third edition. He is coeditor of the *Journal of Rational-Emotive & Cognitive-Behavior Therapy*. He has four children (Matt, Dan, Thomas, and Anna) and two grandchildren (Jack and Elouise). He loves to cook Italian food and makes great risotto, pasta, and pizza.

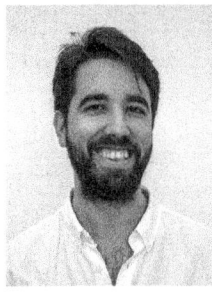

Alexandre Vaz, PhD, is cofounder and chief academic officer of Sentio University, Los Angeles, California. He provides deliberate practice workshops and advanced clinical training and supervision to clinicians around the world. Dr. Vaz is the author/coeditor of multiple books on deliberate practice and psychotherapy training and two series of clinical training books: The Essentials of Deliberate Practice (American Psychological Association) and Advanced Therapeutics, Clinical and Interpersonal Skills (Elsevier). He has held multiple committee roles for the Society for the Exploration of Psychotherapy Integration (SEPI) and the Society for Psychotherapy Research (SPR). Dr. Vaz is founder and host of "Psychotherapy Expert Talks," an acclaimed interview series with distinguished psychotherapists and therapy researchers.

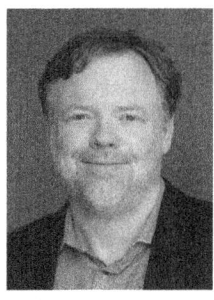

Tony Rousmaniere, PsyD, is cofounder and program director of Sentio University, Los Angeles, California. He provides workshops, webinars, and advanced clinical training and supervision to clinicians around the world. Dr. Rousmaniere is the author/coeditor of multiple books on deliberate practice and psychotherapy training and two series of clinical training books: The Essentials of Deliberate Practice (American Psychological Association) and Advanced Therapeutics, Clinical and Interpersonal Skills (Elsevier). In 2017, he published the widely cited article "What Your Therapist Doesn't Know" in *The Atlantic Monthly.* Dr. Rousmaniere supports the open-data movement and publishes his aggregated clinical outcome data, in deidentified form, on his website (https://drtonyr.com/). A Fellow of APA, he was awarded the Early Career Award by the Society for the Advancement of Psychotherapy (APA Division 29).